Y0-ASD-771

CONSULTING EDITOR

SUZANNE S. PREVOST, PhD, RN, Nursing Professor and National HealthCare Chair of Excellence, Middle Tennessee State University, School for Nursing, Murfreesboro, Tennessee

EDITORIAL BOARD

RUTH KLEINPELL, PhD, RN, FAAN, FAANP, FCCM, Professor, Rush University College of Nursing; Teacher-Practitioner, Rush University Medical Center; and Nurse-Practitioner, Our Lady of the Resurrection Medical Center, Chicago, Illinois

STEPHEN D. KRAU, PhD, RN, CT, Associate Professor of Nursing, Vanderbilt University Medical Center, Nashville, Tennessee

JANE LESKE, PhD, RN, Associate Professor, School of Nursing, University of Wisconsin-Milwaukee, Milwaukee, Wisconsin

CAROL A. RAUEN, MS, RN, CCRN, Instructor, School of Nursing and Health Studies, Georgetown University, Washington, DC

PAMELA RUDISILL, MSN, RN, CCRN, Associate Executive Director of Nursing, Lake Norman Regional Medical Center, Mooresville, North Carolina

MARILYN SAWYER SOMMERS, PhD, RN, FAAN, Professor, College of Nursing, University of Cincinnati, Cincinnati, Ohio

CATHY J. THOMPSON, PhD, RN, CCRN, Assistant Professor, School of Nursing, University of Colorado Health Sciences Center, Denver, Colorado

MARITA TITLER, PhD, RN, FAAN, Director of Nursing Research, Quality and Outcomes Management, Department of Nursing Services, University of Iowa Hospitals and Clinics, Iowa City, Iowa

MICHAEL WILLIAMS, MSN, RN, Assistant Professor, Department of Nursing, Eastern Michigan University, Ypsilanti, Michigan

GUEST EDITOR

STEPHEN D. KRAU, PhD, RN, CT, Associate Professor of Nursing, Vanderbilt University Medical Center, Nashville, Tennessee

CONTRIBUTORS

SHARON BRYANT, MSN, ACNP, Instructor of Nursing, Acute Care Nurse Practitioner Program, Vanderbilt University School of Nursing; Nurse Practitioner, Kindred Hospital, Nashville, Tennessee

FRANCISCA CISNEROS-FARRAR, EdD, RN, Professor and Director, School of Nursing, Austin Peay State University, Clarksville; Staff Nurse, Neurology Intensive Care Unit, St. Thomas Hospital, Nashville, Tennessee

BETH TOWERY DAVIDSON, MSN, RN, ACNP, CCRN, The Heart Group, Nashville, Tennessee

TERRI ALLISON DONALDSON, RN, MN, ACNP, Instructor, Vanderbilt University School of Nursing, Nashville, Tennessee

JOHN TRAVIS DUNLAP, MSN, APRN, BC, Instructor of Nursing, Adult Nurse Practitioner Program, Vanderbilt University School of Nursing, Nashville, Tennessee

BARBARA FOUTS FLICEK, MSN, RN, FNP, Family Nurse Practitioner, Internal Medicine of Newton County, Covington, Georgia

JOAN E. KING, PhD, RNC, ACNP, ANP, Associate Professor and Program Director for Acute Care Nurse Practitioner Program, Vanderbilt University School of Nursing, Nashville, Tennessee

STEPHEN D. KRAU, PhD, RN, CT, Associate Professor of Nursing, Vanderbilt University Medical Center, Nashville, Tennessee

LEIGH ANN McINNIS, PhD, APRN, FNP, Associate Professor, School of Nursing, Middle Tennessee State University, Murfreesboro, Tennessee

KATE MOORE, RN, MSN, CCRN, CEN, ACNP-BC, NREMT-P, Clinical Research Coordinator, Clinical Care Services, Air Evac Lifeteam, Nashville, Tennessee

MARIA OVERSTREET, MSN, RN, CCNS, Assistant Professor of Nursing, Vanderbilt University School of Nursing, Nashville, Tennessee

LYNN C. PARSONS, DSN, RN, CNA-BC, Professor and Director, School of Nursing, Middle Tennessee State University, Murfreesboro, Tennessee

MARIA A. SMITH, DSN, RN, CCRN, COI, Professor, School of Nursing, Middle Tennessee State University, Murfreesboro, Tennessee

TASHA L. SMITH, BA, Interim Director of Research, Tennessee Cardiovascular Research Institute (A Division of The Heart Group, PLLC), Nashville, Tennessee

JENNIFER WILBECK, MSN, ACNP, Assistant Professor, Acute Care Nurse Practitioner Program, Vanderbilt University School of Nursing; Nurse Practitioner, Centennial Medical Center Emergency Department, Nashville, Tennessee

CONTENTS

diagnosis difficult. This difficult diagnostic dilemma warrants an understanding of ticks, their habitats, symptoms of illnesses, and immediate treatment to ameliorate the severity and fatalities caused by these diseases.

This article describes the etiology, symptoms and stages, pathophysiology, diagnosis, treatment, and prevention of Lyme disease and a cluster of similar symptoms called "Southern tick-associated rash illness." It is important for the critical care nurse to be alert to the possibility of these infections because some of the symptoms can have devastating effects on the heart and meninges. In some cases Lyme disease may be a comorbidity, not the primary reason a patient is admitted to an ICU. The cause of the symptoms must be recognized for effective treatment to be initiated.

Critical care nurses care for patients in multisystem failure as a result of trauma and manage infections related to these injuries or medical disorders. This article reviews the role of the critical care nurse in caring for patients who are being treated for infections with varying etiologies. Drug review and classification are presented for antibacterial, antifungal, and antiviral medications, including common side effects, adverse reactions, and toxicity signals. The proactive critical care nurse can save patients' lives, decrease hospital length of stay, and save the hospital fiscal resources that would have gone to treatment of illness complications.

Antimicrobial resistance complicates the approach to patient management in critical care settings. Infections resistant to antimicrobial intervention are a frequent cause of mortality and morbidity in hospitalized patients. Antimicrobial resistance is of particular concern to nurses in critical care units because they administer larger quantities of antimicrobial agents than their counterparts in other parts of the hospital. Mechanisms to prevent and manage this ever-increasing problem are imperative to reduce ramifications that include increased health care costs and increased use of valuable resources.

Whereas methicillin resistant *Staphylococcus aureus* (MRSA) is an ever-increasing endemic nosocomial infection responsible for over 55% of infections in critical care settings, the available treatments are becoming less effective. Nurses need to be equipped with the evidence-based knowledge and tools available to curtail the rise of MRSA infections. This article provides a general overview of MRSA, its evolution, risk factors, disease development, and reviews guidelines for infection control and strategies for culture change.

Although vancomycin-resistant enterococci (VRE) are an increasing threat in critical care areas, the available treatments are not increasing at the same rate. Nurses working in these critical care areas are in a unique position to provide their patients with the care to prevent and treat VRE infections appropriately. This article provides a general overview of VRE, describes its origin, diagnosis, and management, and discusses strategies for surveillance and prevention.

FORTHCOMING ISSUES

RECENT ISSUES

THE CLINICS ARE NOW AVAILABLE ONLINE!

Access your subscription at:
www.theclinics.com

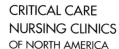
CRITICAL CARE
NURSING CLINICS
OF NORTH AMERICA

ELSEVIER
SAUNDERS

Crit Care Nurs Clin N Am 19 (2007) xi–xii

Preface

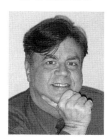

Stephen D. Krau, PhD, RN, CT
Guest Editor

When considering the topic of *infections* in critical care areas, there are many avenues that manuscripts can explore to help the critical care nurse ameliorate the incidence, and to identify infections that occur in critical care areas. Intensive care units (ICUs) have become increasingly important in the last decade as the location where many infections occur. Although the number of acute care beds in hospitals has decreased in the last 20 years, the number of intensive care beds has increased. Patients in ICUs have a higher risk of acquiring infections than patients in noncritical care units. It has been reported that up to 45% of hospital-acquired infections occur in ICU patients, although these patients only occupy 8% of hospital beds [1].

Patients in ICUs with infections can be divided into three distinct groups: (1) those with hospital-acquired infections, (2) those with hospital-acquired infections before they are admitted to the ICU, and (3) those with community-acquired infections. This issue will explore elements of all three populations to varying degrees. Where a complete issue could easily be the focus of each of these groups, it is the hope of the authors that the overview of the immune system will lead the readers to information that they will find particularly important and meaningful.

This issue provides an overview of general infections and their treatments, including bacterial and rickettsial infections. Additionally, there is an overview of infections caused by antibiotic-resistant organisms. These infections have been associated with increased morbidity, expense, and mortality. In the most recent report from the National Nosocomial Infection Surveillance system report, methicillin-resistant *Streptococcus aureus* (MRSA) and vancomycin resistance among entercoccol isolates were both significantly increased compared with the 2002 to 2003 year [2]. The continued emergence and proliferation in the number of antibiotic-resistant isolates from ICUs have made these infections difficult to treat, but imperative to be on the forefront of the care provided by the critical care nurse.

A large portion of this issue is devoted to antimicrobial-resistant organisms. The expanding problem of antimicrobial resistance remains a major public debate. Attention in the lay and medical press is often focused on MRSA as the leading cause of nosocomial infection by antimicrobial-resistant pathogens. We now have MRSA that is acquired in the community, and is not just limited to hospital settings. The rise in MRSA prevalence in health care settings in many parts of the world is increasingly recognized as a serious threat to health [3].

Sepsis and multiple organ dysfunction syndrome (MODS) continue to plague intensivists, as the mortality from these processes has been

0899-5885/07/$ - see front matter © 2007 Elsevier Inc. All rights reserved.
doi:10.1016/j.ccell.2006.11.003

found to be from 30% to 80%. A review of sepsis and MODS will identify current issues surrounding these issues that will help the critical care nurse understand the dynamics, with hopes of earlier interventions to ameliorate the devastating effects of these processes.

The issue ends with the controversial discussion over the possibility of an avian influenza endemic. Although the actual organism of our next endemic provides much controversial discussion, history has shown how these catastrophes emerge, and how preparation for such events impacts patients and health care workers. Clinical and ethical issues are considered, as an endemic will impact critical care nurses not only as professionals, but on a very personal level as well, especially for those of us who are care takers of our own family members. Many aspects of an endemic warrant consideration before it occurs, as relying on one source to ameliorate the effects of any catastrophe involving large numbers of people has not proven effective. One needs only to look at the aftermath of the hurricane Katrina in 2005 for evidence. The strain on the health care system, our economic system, and the alterations in the lives to which we have become accustomed will be altered. So the question is appropriate: Are we ready?

Our course toward all of these issues begins in keeping informed. Through this method we move to other strategies and interventions for our patients and ourselves such as education, feedback, and contributions to processes to control what lies ahead.

Stephen D. Krau, PhD, RN, CT
Associate Professor of Nursing
Vanderbilt University Medical Center
360 Frist Hall, 461 21st Avenue South
Nashville, TN 37240, USA

E-mail address: stephen.krau@vanderbilt.edu

References

[1] Richards M, Thursky K, Buising K. Epidemiology, prevalence and sites of infections in intensive care units. Semin Respir Care Crit Care Med 2003;24(1):3–22.
[2] Smith RL. Prevention of infection in the intensive care unit. Curr Opin Infect Dis 2006;19:323–6.
[3] Cosgrove SE, Carmeli Y. The impact of antimicrobial resistance on health and economic outcomes. Clin Infect Dis 2003;36:1433–7.

Crit Care Nurs Clin N Am 19 (2007) 1–8

Immune Responses to Infection

Terri Allison Donaldson, RN, MN, ACNP

Vanderbilt University School of Nursing, 364 Frist Hall, 461 21st Avenue South, Nashville, TN 37240, USA

Immunity is "the ability of the body to resist almost all types of organisms or toxins that tend to damage tissues and organs" [1]. "Immunity" refers to the body's specific protective response to an invading foreign organism or agent [2]. Invading organisms that cause disease, called "pathogens," include bacteria, viruses, fungi, protozoa, and helminthes (worms) [3,4]. Protozoa and worms usually are classified together as parasites. The immune system also can develop responses to the body's own cells, resulting in autoimmune disease, or against aberrantly developed cancer cells in the body. These foreign invaders are antigens. An antigen is "any substance that can elicit an immune response," and "all living cells have antigens on their cell surfaces" [5]. This article discusses the process whereby the immune system recognizes, becomes activated, and responds to the presence of infectious pathogens in the body. Box 1 defines terms used in this article.

Although the focus of this article is immune responses to infection, the inflammatory response can be activated by noninfectious issues. Inflammation can occur in response to other insults, such as trauma, chemical exposure, myocardial infarction, and malignancies [5].

The primary role of the immune system is to recognize self antigens from non-self antigens [5–7]. Antigens on a person's own body cells are recognized as "self" and are tolerated by the individual's immune system [5]. Non-self antigens are perceived as foreign, and the intact immune system attempts to rid the body of these invaders.

The initial defenses to invasion of a pathogen, or foreign antigen, into the body are the physical barriers of the skin and mucous membranes [3,8]. When these barriers are breached and the pathogen enters the body, the innate and acquired immune systems recognize the pathogen, become activated, and respond to destroy the pathogen.

Initial innate responses may be sufficient to eradicate the organism before infection occurs [3]. In other cases the pathogen is not destroyed, and the acquired immune system events destroy the pathogen. Failure of the innate and acquired immune actions to eradicate the pathogen can result in infection.

The response to infection can be described as two distinct but interrelated stages. Inflammation, involving the innate immune system, occurs initially and is the first line of defense against invading organisms [3]. If the antigen is not destroyed by the actions of the innate immune system, the acquired immune system is triggered. This inflammatory-immune response immune response can be divided into three phases: recognition, activation, and response to activation.

Recognition begins when certain components of the immune system become aware that a foreign antigen is present in the body. The innate immune system is activated and initiates a response to the antigen. If the pathogen is not destroyed, components of the innate defenses process the antigen and present it to the acquired immune system [5]. Once activated, the acquired immune system initiates cellular and humoral responses to rid the body of the foreign invader.

Inflammation

Inflammation occurs as a nonspecific innate immune response that plays a vital role in fighting infection [3,5]. The inflammatory response is initiated by tissue damage at the site of infection, resulting in the release of inflammatory mediators from the injured tissue and by the macrophages

E-mail address: terri.donaldson@vanderbilt.edu

2   DONALDSON

Box 1. Definition of terms

Acquired immunity: An adaptive immune response; the ability of the body to recognize specific antigens as foreign. T lymphocytes become sensitized to an antigen, and B lymphocytes secrete antibodies against the antigen.

Alternative pathway: Activation of the complement system through complement 3

Antibody: A plasma protein produced in response to an antigen that mediates humoral immunity. Immunoglobulin is another name for antibody.

Antigen: A cell marker on the cell surface that allows the body to differentiate self from non-self

Antigen presentation: The process by which certain cells in the body express antigen on the cell surface. Macrophages, dendritic cells, and B cells are professional antigen-presenting cells.

Antigen processing: Conversion of an antigen into a form recognized by lymphocytes

B cells: Lymphocytes developed in the bone marrow and involved in humoral immunity. Their primary function is production of antigen-specific antibodies. They represent 10% to 20% of circulating lymphocytes.

CD markers: Cell surface molecules used to differentiate different cell populations

Chemokines: A large group of cytokines with chemotactic and cell-activating properties

Chemotaxis: Increased directional migration of cells

Classical pathway: The pathway by which antigen-antibody complexes activate complement

Complement: A group of serum proteins that mediate inflammation, activate phagocytes, and lyse cell membranes

Cytokines: Inflammatory molecules produced by macrophages and monocytes; communicate with all leukocytes and other blood cells

Dendritic cells: the most potent antigen-presenting cells

Humoral: Pertaining to extracellular fluids, including serum and lymph

Inflammation: A series of reactions that results in migration of immune molecules to sites of infection or tissue damage

Innate immunity: "Natural immunity," the nonspecific inherent ability to resist antigen invasion, which occurs immediately after pathogen invasion and does not require prior exposure

Interleukins: Groups of molecules in the cytokine family capable of signaling between cells of the immune system

Kinins: Vasoactive mediators produced in response to tissue injury

Opsonization: Coating of antigen to facilitate phagocytosis

Pathogen: An infectious antigen; any microorganism with the potential to cause tissue injury or disease

Phagocyte: A cell capable of phagocytosis

Phagocytosis: the process by which cells engulf and enclose material

T cells: Differentiated from thymus, involved in cellular immunity; comprise 75% of circulating lymphocytes

------

Refs. [3,5,6,9–12,20].

and neutrophils responding to the antigen [3]. Inflammation provides a physical barrier to prevent the spread of infection and to promote the repair of injured tissue [3].

When the pathogen breaks through the body's physical barriers, the macrophages and neutrophils recognize the pathogen as foreign and begin the process of phagocytosis, in which the antigen is engulfed and processed [3,5,9]. Monocytes, located in the circulation, migrate to the site of entry or area of tissue injury and are transformed into tissue macrophages [3]. Polymorphonuclear leukocytes (PMNs) are white blood cells that respond to the antigen. Neutrophils are the primary PMN and are considered the foremost defense against invading microorganisms [3,5]. Basophils and eosinophils are other types of PMNs involved in the innate immune response. Natural killer cells and mast cells have a role in the inflammatory response as well [10]. Table 1 describes each cell's specific activity.

The innate immune response results in physical changes in the area of invasion that typically are associated with inflammation. Inflammatory mediators are released from the injured tissue and by the macrophages and neutrophils responding to the antigen. Inflammatory mediators include histamine, kinins, eicosanoids, complement, and cytokines [5,11,12]. Histamine and the kinins cause vasodilatation and increased capillary permeability at the site of injury. Kinins also stimulate chemotaxis, or movement, of greater numbers of neutrophils into the area. Eicosanoids, such as prostaglandin and thromboxane, induce fever and pain and stimulate platelet aggregation and vasoconstriction to achieve hemostasis [5,11].

Complement is a group of plasma proteins derived from the liver and macrophages that becomes activated directly by the antigen [3]. Activation of complement occurs in a cascade fashion on the surface of the antigen [2,11]. The principle functions of complement are chemotaxis, enhancement of phagocytosis, lysis of the pathogen, release of inflammatory mediators, and triggering of the acquired immune response [2–5,11,12].

Cytokines are inflammatory molecules released predominately by macrophages [13]. Cytokines include tumor necrosis factor and interleukins (IL). IL-6 is a major mediator of acute phase proteins, whereas IL-1 affects the function of other leukocytes [5,13,14]. Table 2 gives a more detailed description of the role of the cytokine inflammatory mediators.

Acute-phase proteins are another type of inflammatory mediator located in the serum. Acute-phase proteins include certain complement factors, C-reactive protein, fibrinogen, and granulocyte colony-stimulating factor [11]. Acute-phase protein serum concentration rises rapidly in response to cytokines, primarily IL-6. C-reactive protein is believed to activate complement and bind with phagocytic cells. Serum levels of C-reactive protein can be monitored to determine the intensity of the inflammatory process [13].

Actions of complement, the cytokines, and other inflammatory mediators cause the signs and symptoms associated with infection. Vasodilatation and increased blood vessel permeability increases local blood flow and promotes leaking of fluid into the area of injury, resulting in heat, redness, and edema in the area of injury [3,5,8,11]. With the increase in vascular permeability, fibrinogen leaks into the intravascular tissue to cause clotting, which helps "wall off" the pathogen and prevent its spread to other areas of the body [5]. Adhesion molecules expressed by injured endothelium cause leukocytes to stick to the walls of the blood vessel. The increase in vascular permeability allows the leukocytes to migrate into the tissue to the site of infection [3]. Migration and actions of the leukocytes, primarily the neutrophils and macrophages, in the inflamed tissue cause pain at the site [3,14]. As a consequence of leukocyte migration into the local area, engulfment, processing, and destruction of the pathogen occur through phagocytosis [3,5,14]. Once the antigen is ingested by the leukocyte, the processed

Table 1
Types of leukocytes

Leukocyte	Function
Polymorphonuclear leukocytes	
Neutrophils	Major leukocytes in bacterial infection
Eosinophils	Recognize parasites and allergens
Basophils	Mediate inflammation
Mononuclear leukocytes	
Monocytes	Circulate in the blood or stored in lymph tissue
Macrophages	Highly phagocytic, transformed from monocytes in the tissue
Lymphocytes—B and T cells	Cells of acquired immune system
Plasma cells	Antibody-secreting B cells
Mast cells	Distributed near blood vessels in tissues, contain inflammatory mediators
Natural killer cells	Nonspecifically kill virally infected cells and tumor cells; an important link between innate and acquired immune systems

Data from Refs. [5,10,12].

Table 2
Inflammatory mediators

Mediator	Source	Action
Histamine	Mast cells, basophils, platelets	Vasodilatation, increased capillary permeability, contraction of bronchial smooth muscle
Kinins (ie, bradykinin)	Generated in plasma	Tissue damage activates Hageman factor Hageman factor activates kallikrein Activated kallikrein catalyzes split of kinins Kinins cause vasodilatation, increase in capillary permeability, chemotaxis of neutrophils, stimulation of pain receptors in injured area

Eicosanoids
  Prostaglandins
  Thromboxanes
  Leukotrienes
	Cellular injury stimulates synthesis of arachidonic acid; enzymes convert to prostaglandins and thromboxanes.
	Leukotrienes synthesized in leukocytes, mast cells, platelets, heart/lung and vascular tissue
		Prostaglandins: prostaglandin E produces sustained vasodilatation, fever-inducing pyrogen, sensitizes pain receptors; prostacyclin inhibits platelet aggregation leading to clot dissolution
		Thromboxanes: thromboxane A induces platelet aggregation, vasoconstriction resulting in hemostasis
		Leukotrienes: enhance inflammation, capillary permeability, chemotaxis, smooth muscle contraction

Complement	Activation:
	Classical pathway: C1 activation by antigen-antibody complexing
	Alternative pathway: activation at C3 level by initiation of plasmin and protease from damaged cells or pathogen
		Opsonization of pathogen enhances phagocytosis by macrophages and neutrophils
		Promotes opsonization of pathogens and enhances phagocytosis by macrophages and neutrophils
		Lysis of pathogen
		Agglutination of pathogen
		Neutralization of toxins from pathogen
		Chemotaxis
		Activation of mast cells and basophils increasing histamine release
		Increased histamine/kinin production:
		  Vasodilatation
		  Increased capillary permeability
		  Coagulation of proteins in tissue spaces

Cytokines		
Tumor necrosis factor	Macrophages Natural killer cells T cells	Enhances inflammation and coagulation; induces fever, sleep, anorexia
IL-1	Macrophages	Lymphocyte activation; induces fever; enhances inflammation and coagulation; stimulates production other cytokines
IL-2	Helper T cells	T-cell proliferation/differentiation; induces cytokine production by T cells; enhances natural killer cells
IL-3	T cells	Growth/differentiation of all bone marrow stem cell lines
IL-4	T cells	B-cell growth factor
IL-5	T cells	B-cell growth/differentiation
IL-6	T and B cells Macrophages Fibroblasts	B-cell growth/differentiation into plasma cells; induces acute phase proteins
Lymphotoxin	T and B cells Macrophages Mast cells	Lysis of some target cells; PMN activation
Acute-phase proteins	Liver	Found in serum; levels rise rapidly during infection or inflammation; has proinflammatory effects. Measurement of levels may reflect intensity of inflammatory process. Example is C-reactive protein.

Data from Refs. [5,12].

material, in the form of peptides or protein fragments, is expressed on the surface of the leukocyte, creating an antigen-presenting cell, whose role is to activate the acquired immune response [3,5,9].

Activation of the acquired immune system

The inflammatory process mediated by the innate immune system may result in destruction of the microorganism. If the antigen persists in the body despite inflammatory efforts, the acquired immune system is activated and responds to eliminate the pathogen. The steps of this acquired immune response are shown in Fig. 1.

Recognition and activation

Antigen-presenting cells are the link between the innate and the adaptive immune systems [12]. Tissue macrophages and dendritic cells, another type of phagocyte, are professional antigen-presenting cells that present antigen fragments to T

lymphocytes of the cellular immune system and to B lymphocytes of the humoral immune system [6,9,12,15,16]. This antigen presentation usually occurs in a lymph node adjacent to the site of pathogen invasion [5]. Antigen-presenting cells containing antigen fragments release cytokine and IL-1, which in turn activate T lymphocytes [17]. The invading antigen itself directly activates B lymphocytes [5,18].

Cellular immune response to activation

Once activated by the antigen-presenting cells and IL-1, helper T lymphocytes (also known as "CD4 cells") are activated and release interleukins [4,19]. Interleukins, especially IL-2, activate and differentiate the different types of T lymphocytes and initiate the B-lymphocyte response [5,20,21]. Cytotoxic T lymphocytes (also known as "CD8" cells or "killer T cells") respond to lyse the pathogen that has invaded the cells in the body by creating fenestrations in the cell. Water enters

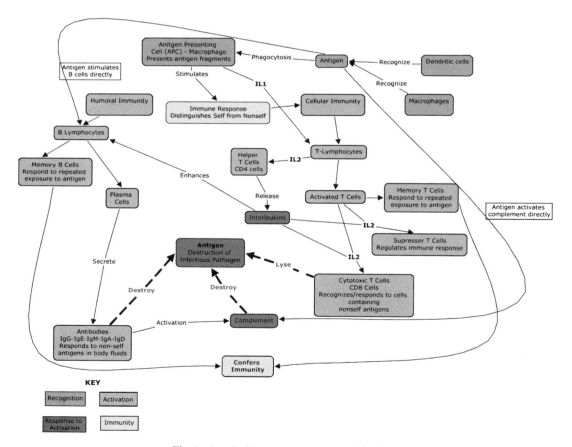

Fig. 1. Acquired immune responses to infection.

the infected cell so that the cell bursts and is destroyed [5]. IL-2 also stimulates proliferation of other helper and cytotoxic T lymphocytes to maintain the immune response until the pathogen is eliminated. Suppressor T lymphocytes function to "turn off" the immune reaction to prevent harm to normal tissue in the body by the activated immune response [2,5]. Memory T lymphocytes remain in the lymph system and result in long-lasting immunity to the pathogen [2,5].

Humoral immune response to activation

Activated B lymphocytes respond by growing, proliferating, and differentiating into plasma cells and memory cells [5,9,18,22,23]. Plasma cells, derived from B cells, secrete antibodies, such as IgG, that respond to and destroy pathogens in the body fluids [5,18]. Complement, activated by direct encounter with the antigen and by the antibody-secreting plasma cells, also destroys the pathogen. Like memory T cells, memory B lymphocytes are stored in lymph tissue and can respond rapidly to subsequent exposure to the same antigen. Memory B and T lymphocytes are the cells that confer immunity and activate the immune response with repeated exposure to the antigen [3,5,18,21].

Summary

The inflammatory and immune response to infection is a complex physiologic process targeted at removing foreign invaders, or pathogens, from the body. The initial inflammation that occurs may eliminate the pathogen, so that no infection results. If the inflammatory response is insufficient to remove the pathogen from the body, the acquired immune system becomes activated, stimulating the actions of T and B lymphocytes, which also attempt to eradicate the infectious pathogen. If this activity is successful, the body remains free of infection. If the pathogen remains viable in the body despite inflammatory and immune system actions, active infection ensues. The severity of the infection and the body's response depend on a multitude of factors including intactness of barrier defenses, immune competence of the host, virulence of the invading organism, and other underlying disease processes at work in the body. The critical care nurse must understand the inflammatory and immune responses to infection to appreciate the local and systemic effects of infection in the body and the rationale for treatment modalities.

References

[1] Guyton AC, Hall JE. Resistance of the body to infection: II immunity and allergy. In: Guyton AC, Hall JE, editors. Textbook of medical physiology. 10th edition. Philadelphia: Saunders; 2000. p. 402–12.

[2] Williams PE. Fundamental immunology. 5th edition. Philadelphia: Lippincott Williams & Wilkins; 2003.

[3] Janeway CA, Travers P, Walport M, et al. Immunobiology: the immune system in health and disease. 5th edition. Oxford (UK): Taylor & Francis; 2001. Available at: http://www.ncbi.nlm.nih.gov/entrez/query.fcgidb=Books&cmd = search&term=charles+janeway. Accessed September 28, 2006.

[4] Hunt R. Microbiology and immunology on-line. 2006. Available at: http://www.med.sc.edu/micro/book/immunol-sta.htm. Accessed July 28, 2006.

[5] Lancaster LE. Physiology of inflammation and immunity. In: Lancaster LE, editor. Core curriculum for nephrology nursing. 4th edition. Pitman (NJ): American Nephrology Nurses' Association; 2001. p. 33–55.

[6] Crow MK. Costimulatory molecules and T-cell-B-cell interactions. Rheum Dis Clin North Am 2004; 30:175–91.

[7] Sayegh MH, Vella JP. MHC structure and function. Up to Date Online 2003. Available at: http://www.uptodateonline.com. Accessed August 20, 2003.

[8] Opal SM, Keusch GT. Host responses to infection. In: Cohen J, Powderly WG, editors. Infectious diseases. 2nd edition. Philadelphia: Mosby; 2004. Available at: http://home.mdconsult.com/das/book/body/496662626/1209/9.html. Accessed July 28, 2006.

[9] Call ME, Wucherpfennig KW. Antigen presenting cells. Up to Date Online 2006. Available at: http://www.uptodateonline.com. Accessed July 28, 2006.

[10] Fleisher TA, Oliveira JB. Functional and molecular evaluation of lymphocytes. J Allergy Clin Immunol 2004;114:227–34.

[11] Parslow TG, Bainton DF. Innate immunity. In: Parslow TG, Sites DP, Terr AI, et al editors. Medical immunology. 10th edition. Available at: http://online.statref.com. Accessed August 14, 2006.

[12] Male D, Bristoff J, Roth DB, et al. Immunology. 7th edition. Philadelphia: Mosby; 2006.

[13] Kushner I. Acute phase proteins. Up to Date Online 2006; Available at: http://www.uptodateonline.com. Accessed July 28, 2006.

[14] Sibbald WJ, Neviere R. Pathophysiology of sepsis. Up to Date Online 2006. Available at: http://www.uptodateonline.com. Accessed July 28, 2006.

[15] Bonilla FA. The cellular immune response. Up to Date Online 2005. Available at: http://www.uptodateonline.com.Accessed September 6, 2005.

[16] Calandra T, Holland SM. Infections in the immunocompromised host. In: Parslow TG, Stites DP, Terr AI, et al editors. Medical immunology. 10th

edition. Available at: http://online.statref.com. Accessed July 28, 2006.

[17] Steinke JW, Borish L. Cytokines and chemokines. J Allergy Clin Immunol 2006;117:S441–5.

[18] Weinstein E, Peeva E, Putterman C, et al. B-cell biology. Rheum Dis Clin North Am 2004;30: 159–74.

[19] Seely RR, Stephens TD, Tate P. Anatomy and physiology. 7th edition. Boston: McGraw Hill; 2006.

[20] MacConmara M, Lederer JA. B cells. Crit Care Med 2005;33:S514–6.

[21] Vallejo AN, Davila E, Weyand CM, et al. Biology of T lymphocytes. Rheum Dis Clin North Am 2004;30: 135–57.

[22] Bonilla FA. The humoral immune response. Up to Date Online 2005. Available at: http://www. uptodateonline.com. Accessed September 6, 2005.

[23] Sommers MS. The cellular basis of septic shock. Crit Care Nurs Clin North Am March 2003;15:13–25.

ELSEVIER
SAUNDERS

Crit Care Nurs Clin N Am 19 (2007) 9–15

CRITICAL CARE
NURSING CLINICS
OF NORTH AMERICA

An Anatomy of an Infection: Overview of the Infectious Process

Kate Moore, RN, MSN, CCRN, CEN, ACNP-BC, NREMT-P

Clinical Care Services, Air Evac Lifeteam, 4502 Glendale Place, Nashville, TN 37215, USA

The immune system is a complex network of protection, offense and defense. The protection includes intact skin, cleanliness, and avoidance of exposure with personal protective equipment. The offense is a strong, intact immune system; the defense is both internal and external. The internal defense system is an immune system that mobilizes against invaders, and the external defense system is adjunctive to immune system. There are physiologic reserves and blockades to prevent and minimize infections. The formation of the immune system begins early in life, and the immune system serves throughout maturity. As with many other physiologic systems, the immune system begins to fail with age or when taxed.

Preventing infections has a long tradition in the profession of nursing. During the Crimean War, Florence Nightingale laid out the guidelines of washing hands, keeping skin intact, practicing good hygiene, and allowing the patient fresh air and sunshine [1]. Prevention has advanced with the advent of immunizations and vaccines. From Edward Jenner's introduction of smallpox vaccine in 1796 to the recent introduction of the human Papillomavirus vaccine, scientists have sought methods of enhancing the immune system and preventing infection [2].

Immune system physiology

A review of the anatomy and physiology of the immune system and the immune response is essential to understanding "the anatomy of an infection." Anatomically, the immune system is comprised of the lymphoid organs and tissues.

The lymphoid organs include the lymph nodes, thymus, spleen, tonsils, and the mucosa-associated lymphoid tissue. The lymphoid tissue is composed of lymphocytes and plasma concentrated in the gastrointestinal tract and bone marrow but present throughout the body. The human body functions well in the absence of the tonsils and spleen, and with age the thymus shrinks. The role of the thymus is most important in childhood and in the initial development of lymphocytes and childhood immunity. The lymph nodes and lymphoid tissue are critically important to the function of the immune system. In some cases of exaggerated immune response (eg, metastatic cancer), portions of the lymph nodes may be removed [3,4].

The cells of the immune system include B lymphocytes, T lymphocytes, natural killer cells, immunoglobulins, and macrophages; processes include formation of specific antibodies and antigen and immunogen or hapten recognition. The T and B lymphocytes are considered the only immunocompetent cells. They detect specific antigens as specific lymphocytes initiate the action of immunity. The development of immunity is a function of T and B cells as well as the interaction of macrophages with antigens. This interaction results in the function known as "immune surveillance," the protection of the human organism from microorganisms, diseases, and foreign tissue [5–7]. Through the process of immune surveillance, antigens are detected and eliminated [8].

The B lymphocytes are responsible for immunoglobulin-mediated immunity. These cells originate in the bone marrow and are capable of proliferating and differentiating into memory cells or plasma cells when exposed to an antigen. Plasma cells secrete specific immunoglobulins,

E-mail address: moorekate@air-evac.com

and memory cells are responsible for the storage of a specific clone of B lymphocytes. This storage enables the body to provide immediate production of the antigen-specific immunoglobulin when it is exposed to a specific antigen. These immunoglobulins are referred to as "antibodies."

There are five classes of immunoglobulins: IgM, IgG, IgA, IgE, and IgD. Each of these immunoglobulins has specific characteristics and functions and has a responsibility in host defense and antibody response to infection.

IgM is a macroglobulin and is the largest of the immunoglobulins. It is the first antibody formed in the primary response to antigens. IgM is responsible for mediating cytotoxic responses and can produce antigen–antibody complexes. It reacts efficiently with both bacteria and viruses. IgM levels normally are elevated for about a week during the immune response as it prepares for IgG activity [8–11].

IgG is the major antibody found in the secondary response to antigens. It is the most common antibody found in response to an infection and is the most long-lived. IgG also diffuses across the placental barrier to provide the fetus with passive immunity until the infant can produce an adequate immune defense [9–11].

IgA provides defense against pathogens that attack on exposed surfaces of the body, especially the respiratory tract and the gastrointestinal tract. Secretory IgA is found in saliva, sweat, tears, mucous, bile, and colostrum. IgA is critical in preventing the entry of microorganisms through portals of entry [9–11].

IgE is associated with allergy and anaphylaxis. It is involved in reactions seen in immediate hypersensitivity. When IgE comes in contact with an antigen, it triggers the release of mast cell granulocytes. The release of these mast cell granulocytes causes the body to produce signs and symptoms of allergy and anaphylaxis. High serum levels of IgE are seen in allergy-prone individuals and in certain parasitic infections [9–11].

IgD is the least-understood immunoglobulin. It is found with IgM on the surface of B lymphocytes. The exact function of IgD is not known. Elevated levels of IgD are seen in chronic infections, but the immunoglobulin has no apparent affinity for any particular antigen [9–11].

T lymphocytes provide long-term immunity to the body. They are thought to originate from stem cells in the bone marrow and in the thymus gland. T lymphocytes live in the lymph nodes and spleen. When the T cell encounters a specific antigen, it creates a clone of T cells that can destroy the antigen [11].

T lymphocytes recognize major histocompatibility complex (MHC). The T cell learns to recognize the body's own MHC and develops a strong reaction to foreign MHC. As a result, the T cells become the primary defender against infection or transplanted tissue [12,13].

T cells generally are placed in three categories: killer cells, helper T cells, and suppressor T cells. Killer cells are cytotoxic to foreign cells. They directly kill the invading cell and are essential in killing virally infected cells [14]. Helper T cells work in conjunction with the B lymphocytes. They stimulate the B cell to differentiate into antibody producers. The IgA immunoglobulin response is most dependent on T cells. Helper T cells also interact with phagocytes to enhance the destruction of pathogens [13]. Suppressor T cells control the production of immunoglobulins, either by regulating the proliferation of B cells or by inhibiting the activity of helper T cells.

Macrophages engulf and then digest cellular debris and pathogens either as stationary or mobile cells. They also stimulate lymphocytes and other immune cells to respond to the pathogen. Tissue macrophages are part of a network of phagocytic cells throughout the body. The name of each macrophage reflects its location. Those in the blood are circulating blood monocytes, Kupffer's cells are in the liver, the intraglomerular mesangial cells are found in the kidney; and alveolar macrophages are in lung tissue. Serosal macrophages wander throughout the body as scavengers. The brain microglia are macrophages specific to the brain tissue and enter the brain about the time of birth. Two lymph organs contain macrophages: the spleen contains spleen sinus macrophages, and the lymph node contains lymph node sinus macrophages [11,15].

Most antigens have the property of immunogenicity or stimulate an immune response when they are present. Some molecules become antigenic only when they are with a carrier. These carrier substances are too small to elicit an immune response and are referred to as "haptens." Contact allergens, some drugs, dust particles, dander, chemicals, and poisons are all examples of haptens [4,8,16].

Immunity can be divided into two types of responses: humoral immunity and cell-mediated immunity. Humoral immunity is the immunity afforded the body by B cells and immunoglobulin. It is subdivided further into primary and secondary responses. The primary response occurs when an antigen enters the body: the antibodies begin to build, and after about 6 days antigen-specific antibodies are found in the blood. IgM is the first measurable immunoglobulin and is followed by IgG in about 10 days. The secondary response differs in that the specific antibody production begins almost immediately. Both T and B memory cells are involved in the secondary response [4,10,17]. Cell-mediated immunity refers to T-cell and macrophage-related immunity.

Pathophysiology of immunodeficiency

There are several routes by which the immune system may become deficient and unable to protect the body appropriately. The routes include primary immunodeficiency and secondary immunodeficiency. Secondary immunodeficiency can be placed in two large categories: disease states and iatrogenic causes. In disease states, some portion of the immune system is depressed or decreased in function. Secondary immunodeficiency is seen most frequently in the disease states including diabetes mellitus, disseminated tuberculosis, malignancies, malnutrition, uremia, and viral infections, including HIV infection. The iatrogenic causes include corticosteroid therapy, immunosuppressive therapy to include radiotherapy, and splenectomy [18].

Primary immunodeficiency results from failure of an essential part of the immune system to develop. Humoral immunodeficiencies generally are a pathophysiologic defect in the immune system resulting in either improper immunoglobulin synthesis or immunoglobulin deficiency. Humoral immunodeficiencies may be seen at any time during the human life cycle. The T cells also may incur a pathophysiologic defect, which usually manifests in infancy or childhood [18].

The best-known and most prevalent of the immunodeficiencies is that caused by HIV, the virus that causes AIDS. The virus is spread by body fluid contact, including sexual activity, blood-to-blood contact, and maternal–fetal contact. The epidemiology of HIV is continually changing. In the 1980s the male homosexuals and intravenous-drug users were the populations most affected. Through education and programs such as needle exchanges, the number of new cases in these groups has continued to diminish. There has been a significant increase in HIV in the sexually active heterosexual population. The virus

is known to mutate, and a variety of drug-resistant strains exist. HIV and AIDS represent the largest segment of immunodeficiencies, and the treatment of these conditions is a separate specialty [19–23].

Hypersensitive immune response and autoimmune disease pathophysiology

There are four types of tissue injury caused by hypersensitivity. Type I is immediate hypersensitivity and generally is characterized by an anaphylactic reaction. Examples include anaphylaxis, anaphylactic shock, bronchial asthma, and atopic eczema. Anaphylaxis manifests with an acute reaction usually associated with a wheal-and-flare type skin reaction and vasodilatation. Atopy is also called "allergy" and is the most common of the immediate hypersensitivity reactions. Type II cytotoxic hypersensitivity is seen in hemolytic reactions and in reactions that cause the destruction of specific target cells. Disease examples include Goodpasture's syndrome, myasthenia gravis, and Grave's disease. Type III reactions are manifested in immune complex diseases such as rheumatoid arthritis, systemic lupus erythematous, polyarteritis, cutaneous vasculitis, and fibrosing alveolitis. Type IV reactions are cell-mediated hypersensitivity reactions and include delayed hypersensitivity, granulomatous hypersensitivity response, and contact dermatitis. Transplant or graft rejections also fall into the category of hypersensitivity reactions [17,20,24–28].

Current trends in immunology

Immunology is an evolving science in which new discoveries occur frequently. Through the investigation of one disease process, patterns associated with other diseases and novel ways in which the immune responds are discovered. This section examines a few of the reviews summarizing the new findings in immunology and infectious diseases.

A French study examined nonconventional primary immunodeficiencies and conventional primary immunodeficiencies to examine similarities and differences between the two. Conventional primary immunodeficiencies typically are seen as rare conditions with detectable immunologic abnormalities. Casanova and colleagues [29] described nonconventional primary immunodeficiencies as Mendelian conditions appearing as a narrow susceptibility to infections in otherwise healthy patients. The findings suggest these Mendelian primary immunodeficiencies are more common in the general population than previously thought and might affect children who have a single infectious, allergic, or autoimmune disease.

Tosi [30] reviewed innate immune responses to infection and described the manner in which the innate immune response defends against infection in an effort to provide the host with the time to mobilize the more slowly developing adaptive immunity to protect against subsequent challenges. This response enables the human host to survive many infectious challenges.

Martins and colleagues [31] reviewed the immunologic changes that occur with aging as they relate to transplantation. Many complex changes and remodeling occur in the immune system as the host ages. The age of both the donor and recipient should be considered in transplantation. Advanced age in either should be considered an independent risk factor for poor patient outcomes and graft survival rates.

Marchant and Goldman [32] provide a controversial perspective on immunizations given in childhood to enhance the immune system. Although many groups now are voicing concerns about vaccines in children, the authors suggest administering vaccines even earlier in life to induce protective T-cell–mediated immune responses. Although the authors acknowledge that there are few studies of T-cell–mediated immunity in human newborns and infants, the notion that infections with intracellular pathogens often are more severe or more prolonged in young infants is well supported. This difference suggests that T-cell–mediated immune responses are different in early life.

A German review by Kamradt and Volkmer-Engert [33] examined the mechanisms that trigger autoaggressive attacks by the immune system. Previous clinical and epidemiologic observations suggested a link between infection and autoimmunity. A popular hypothesis considers autoimmunity as a side effect of antimicrobial immune response. T cells with cross-reactive properties, capable of recognizing both microbial and self-peptides, are the prime suspects in the autoaggressive attacks. Each of these T cells can recognize large numbers of different ligands, molecules that attach to receptors as a way of cytoplasmic signaling in a cell. A careful review of the data suggests that the T-cell cross-reactivity is too simple an explanation. It now is thought that a variety of different molecular mechanisms dictate the immunologic outcome of ligand recognition by T cells.

Hygiene hypothesis

Christen and von Herrath [34] reviewed the complex relationship between infections and autoimmunity. The hygiene hypothesis suggests that cleaner living conditions will lead to a greater incidence of autoimmune disorders, asthma, and allergies. Studies of this hypothesis are difficult to perform in human models, so the authors looked predominately to relevant animal models. This review provides a fertile ground for future prospective studies to explore the molecular details of infections and autoimmunity.

Kamradt and colleagues [35] also reviewed the literature as it relates to the hygiene hypothesis and found that infections or exposure to non-pathogenic bacteria may protect individuals from developing some autoimmune and atopic disorders. The literature strongly suggests the current rise in autoimmune and atopic disorders results from a lack of exposure to infections that normally keep the immune system balanced by inducing immunoregulation. The hygiene hypothesis holds great promise as an explanation of the increase in allergies and autoimmune disorders seen today.

Sepsis

Hospital infections have the potential to become life threatening if they progress to sepsis and multiorgan failure. Vodovotz and colleagues [36] reviewed the nature of trauma and infections that elicit an acute inflammatory response. When the acute inflammatory response becomes severe, it may result in pathologic manifestations of sepsis and multiorgan failure or dysfunction. In a review of more than 250 trials, only activated protein C was shown to be useful in modulating inflammation in sepsis. In the review the investigators found a good likelihood that mathematical modeling can provide a means to synthesize in vitro and in vivo data into system-level analytic models of the acute inflammatory response. By simulating these various methods researchers can gain insight into the pathophysiology of the acute inflammatory response, possibly leading to better design of clinical trials in sepsis and trauma.

Marshall and colleagues [37] reviewed methods of source-control management of sepsis. Their primary finding was that source control is a key component in successful sepsis treatment.

Although source control may seem to be one of the most obvious methods of sepsis management, it also is one of the most difficult in which to perform randomized clinical trials.

Cohen and colleagues [38] examined guidelines from 2003 related to management and diagnosis of infection in sepsis for the bedside clinician. Their review pointed out that obtaining a precise bacteriologic diagnosis before starting antibiotic therapy is important for the success of therapeutic strategy during sepsis. The recommendation that two or three blood cultures be performed, preferably on samples taken from a peripheral vein, without interval between samples to avoid delaying therapy, remains a strong component of the diagnostic procedure. When possible, a quantitative approach is preferred in most cases, especially for catheter-related infections and ventilator-associated pneumonia. The review also supports the taking of appropriate samples from soft tissue and intra-abdominal infections. The use of cultures obtained through drains and central lines are discouraged.

Predicting infections in critically ill trauma patients

Patients admitted with trauma injuries generally are at a great risk for infections because of the nature of the injury. The body's first line of defense, the skin, is compromised, and trauma wounds are exposed to all the environmental elements that exist at the location in which the traumatic incident occurred. Gunshot wounds have additional debris and dirt and clothing fibers embedded in the wound if the projectile penetrated the clothing first. Wounds of victims of motor vehicle crashes contain dirt, asphalt, glass, and any other substances that might be present on the street and in the vehicle where the crash occurred. Trauma researchers continue to discover predictors of outcomes in critically ill trauma patients. An area of major concern is the prediction of infection. Albumin and glucose levels have been identified as two variables that may be predictive of outcomes in critically ill trauma patients.

Sung and colleagues [39] looked at serum albumin on admission as a predictor of outcomes in critically ill trauma patients. In a prospective daily data collection involving 1023 patients over a 2-year period, subjects were stratified by serum albumin level on admission, age, gender, injury severity, and comorbid conditions. The outcome was measured by ICU and hospital length of stay, ventilator days, incidence of infection, and mortality. The study found that an admission serum albumin level lower than 2.6 g/dL is a significant independent predictor of morbidity and mortality in trauma patients. Even more predictive is the combination of increased age and low albumin level. The investigators recommend considering early nutrition these high-risk patients.

Hyperglycemia has been linked to outcomes in critically ill trauma patients. At the Baltimore Shock Trauma Center, Sung and colleagues [40] found that admission hyperglycemia (>200 mg/dL) was predictive of outcome in critically ill trauma patients. They found with 25% of 1003 trauma patients demonstrated hyperglycemia on admission. Patients who had hyperglycemia had a significantly greater infection rate (52% versus 32%). The hyperglycemic group had a significantly greater incidence of site-specific infection, specifically respiratory, genitourinary, bloodstream, and skin/wound infections. The study demonstrated that admission hyperglycemia is associated with increased morbidity and mortality in a critically ill general trauma population.

Bochicchio and colleagues [41] monitored persistent hyperglycemia in critically ill trauma patients and found that mortality and morbidity are significantly greater in this population than in those who are not hyperglycemic. The study reviewed prospective data on 942 consecutive trauma patients who had pre-existing diabetes mellitus and who were admitted to the ICU over a 2-year period. Serum glucose levels were monitored on a daily basis and stratified as low, medium, or high glucose. Because hyperglycemia has long been associated with a more critically ill patient, it remains unclear if the hyperglycemia is the actual cause of the worse outcome in the critically ill or is simply a marker of a more critically ill patient.

Predictors of mortality in patients presenting to the emergency department with infection

Patients presenting in emergency departments with infection-related diagnoses are at great risk for mortality and severe morbidity. Shapiro and colleagues [42] performed a prospective cohort study in an urban, academic medical center with 50,000 annual emergency department visits and enrolled 1278 patients over an 8-month period.

In this study, serum lactate was measured as a potential indicator associated with increased mortality in patients presenting to emergency departments with infection. The main outcome measures were all causes of in-hospital mortality in a 28-day period and death within 3 days of presentation to the emergency department. In this group of patients who had signs and symptoms suggesting infection, the level of serum venous lactate was a promising risk-stratification tool.

Summary

The immune system remains an enigmatic system in that each discovery leads to more questions and speculation. It is essential for the critical care nurse to understand the basic physiology that occurs in infections to address the issues in patients in an efficient and timely manner. Thorough patient assessment helps determine predictors and priorities. Although the protective barrier of an intact integument system often is identified as the first and best line of defense against infections, this defense can be strengthened by a critical care nurse who is equipped with the knowledge and understanding of the immune system, the latest research, and the dynamics that ensue within the patient.

References

[1] F. Nightingale Notes on nursing. London: Harrison and Sons; 1859. Reprinted New York: Dover Publications; 1969.

[2] Wikipedia Contributors. Timeline of Vaccines. Available at: http://en.wickipedia.org/wiki/Timeline_of_vaccines. Accessed July 8, 2006.

[3] Bullock BL. Normal immunologic response. In: Bullock BL, editor. Pathophysiology: adaptations and alterations in function. 4th edition. Philadelphia: Lippincott; 1996.

[4] Guyten AC, Hall JE. Textbook of medical physiology. 10th edition. Philadelphia: WB Saunders; 2000.

[5] Beverly P. Tumour immunology. In: Roitt I, Brostoff J, Male D, editors. Immunology. 3rd edition. St. Louis (MO): Mosby; 1993. p. 17.1–17.12.

[6] Greenberg PD. Mechanisms of tumor immunology. In: Stiles DP, Terr AI, Parslow TG, editors. Basic and clinical immunology. 8th edition. Norwalk (CT): Appleton and Lange; 1994. p. 569–77.

[7] Ziegler JL. Cancer in the immunocompromised host. In: Stiles DP, Terr AI, Parslow TG, editors. Basic and clinical immunology. 8th edition. Norwalk (CT): Appleton and Lange; 1994. p. 578–87.

[8] Goodman JW. The immune response. In: Stiles DP, Terr AI, Parslow TG, editors. Basic and clinical immunology. 8th edition. Norwalk (CT): Appleton and Lange; 1994. p. 40–9.

[9] Goodman JW, Parslow TG. Immunoglobulin proteins. In: Stiles DP, Terr AI, Parslow TG, editors. Basic and clinical immunology. 8th edition. Norwalk (CT): Appleton and Lange; 1994. p. 69–79.

[10] Cormack DH. Essential histology. Philadelphia: Lippincott; 1993.

[11] Parslow TG. Lymphocytes and lymphoid tissue. In: Stiles DP, Terr AI, Parslow TG, editors. Basic and clinical immunology. 8th edition. Norwalk (CT): Appleton and Lange; 1994. p. 22–39.

[12] Imboden JB. T lymphocytes and natural killer cells. In: Stiles DP, Terr AI, Parslow TG, editors. Basic and clinical immunology. 8th edition. Norwalk (CT): Appleton and Lange; 1994. p. 94–104.

[13] Male D, Roitt I. Introduction to the immune system. In: Roitt I, Brostoff J, Male D, editors. Immunology. 3rd edition. St. Louis (MO): Mosby; 1993. p. 1.1–1.12.

[14] Herold BC. Virus-host interactions. In: Shulman ST, Phair JP, Sommers HM, editors. The biologic and clinical basis of infectious diseases. 4th edition. Philadelphia: W B Saunders; 1992. p. 36–48.

[15] Lydyard P, Grossi C. Cells involved in immune response. In: Roitt I, Brostoff J, Male D, editors. Immunology. 3rd edition. St. Louis (MO): Mosby; 1993. p. 2.2–2.20.

[16] Coico R, Sunshine G, Benjamini E. Immunology: a short course. 5th edition. New York: Wiley-Liss; 2003.

[17] Kumar V, Fausto N, Abbas A. Robbins and Cotran pathologic basis of disease. 7th edition. Philadelphia: W B Saunders; 2004.

[18] Widmann FK, Itatani CA. An introduction to clinical immunology and serology. 2nd edition. Philadelphia: F A Davis; 1998.

[19] Shilts R. And the band played on. New York: Penguin; 1988.

[20] Damjanov I, Linder J, Anderson WAD, editors. Anderson's pathology. 10th edition. St. Louis (MO): Mosby; 1996.

[21] Mudge-Grout CL. Immunologic disorders. St. Louis (MO): Mosby Yearbook; 1992.

[22] Sepulveda J, Fineberg H, Mann J, editors. AIDS prevention through education: a world view. New York: Oxford University Press; 1992.

[23] Volberding PA, Saag MS. Clinical spectrum of HIV disease. In: DeVita VT, Hellman S, Rosenberg SA, editors. AIDS: etiology, diagnosis, treatment, and prevention. 4th edition. Philadelphia: Lippincott; 1997. p. 203–14.

[24] Roitt I. Autoimmunity and autoimmune disease. In: Roitt I, Brostoff J, Male D, editors. Immunology. 3rd edition. St. Louis (MO): Mosby; 1993.

[25] Steinberg AD. Mechanisms of disordered immune regulation. In: Stiles DP, Terr AI, Parslow TG,

editors. Basic and clinical immunology. 8th edition. Norwalk (CT): Appleton and Lange; 1994. p. 380–6.

[26] Terr AI. Cell-mediated hypersensitivity diseases. In: Stiles DP, Terr AI, Parslow TG, editors. Basic and clinical immunology. 8th edition. Norwalk (CT): Appleton and Lange; 1994. p. 363–70.

[27] Terr AI. Immune-complex allergic diseases. In: Stiles DP, Terr AI, Parslow TG, editors. Basic and clinical immunology. 8th edition. Norwalk (CT): Appleton and Lange; 1994. p. 357–62.

[28] Terr AI. Mechanisms of hypersensitivity. In: Stiles DP, Terr AI, Parslow TG, editors. Basic and clinical immunology. 8th edition. Norwalk (CT): Appleton and Lange; 1994. p. 314–26.

[29] Casanova JL, Fieschi C, Bustamante J, et al. From idiopathic infectious disease to novel primary immunodeficiencies. J Allergy Clin Immunol 2005;116(2): 423–5.

[30] Tosi M. Innate immune responses to infection. J Allergy Clin Immunol 2005;116(2):241–9.

[31] Martins PN, Pratschke J, Pascher A, et al. Age and immune response in organ transplantation. Transplantation 2005;79(2):127–32.

[32] Marchant A, Goldman M. T cell-mediated immune responses in human newborns: ready to learn? Clin Exp Immunol 2005;141(1):10–8.

[33] Kamradt T, Volkmer-Engert R. Cross-reactivity of T lymphocytes in infection and autoimmunity. Mol Divers 2004;8(3):271–80.

[34] Christen U, von Herrath MG. Infections and autoimmunity—good or bad? J Immunol 2005;174(12): 7481–6.

[35] Kamradt T, Goggel R, Erb KJ. Induction, exacerbation and inhibition of allergic and autoimmune diseases by infection. Trends Immunol 2005;26(5): 260–7.

[36] Vodovotz Y, Clermont G, Chow C, et al. Mathematical models of the acute inflammatory response. Curr Opin Crit Care 2004;10(5):383–90.

[37] Marshall JC, Maier RV, Jimenez M, et al. Source control in the management of severe sepsis and septic shock: an evidence-based review. Crit Care Med 2004;32(11 Suppl):S513–26.

[38] Cohen J, Brun-Buisson C, Torres A, et al. Diagnosis of infection in sepsis: an evidence-based review. Crit Care Med 2004;32(11 Suppl):S466–94.

[39] Sung J, Bochicchio GV, Joshi M, et al. Admission serum albumin is predictive of outcome in critically ill trauma patients. Am Surg 2004;70(12):1099–102.

[40] Sung J, Bochicchio GV, Joshi M, et al. Admission hyperglycemia is predictive of outcome in critically ill trauma patients. J Trauma 2005;59(1):80–3.

[41] Bochicchio GV, Sung J, Joshi M, et al. Persistent hyperglycemia is predictive of outcome in critically ill trauma patients. J Trauma 2005;58(5):921–4.

[42] Shapiro NI, Howell MD, Talmor D, et al. Serum lactate as a predictor of mortality in emergency department patients with infection. Ann Emerg Med 2005; 45(5):524–8.

ELSEVIER
SAUNDERS

Crit Care Nurs Clin N Am 19 (2007) 17–26

CRITICAL CARE
NURSING CLINICS
OF NORTH AMERICA

Bacterial Infections: Management by Acute and Critical Care Nurses

Lynn C. Parsons, DSN, RN, CNA-BC[a],*,
Stephen D. Krau, PhD, RN, CT[b,c]

[a]School of Nursing, Box #81, Middle Tennessee State University, Murfreesboro, TN 37132, USA
[b]School of Nursing, Vanderbilt University, 461 21st Avenue South, Nashville, TN 37240, USA
[c]Critical Care Unit, Vanderbilt University Medical Center, 345 Frist Hall, 461 21st Avenue South,
Nashville, TN 37240, USA

Treating bacterial infections is commonplace in United States hospitals. Up to 10% of people admitted to hospitals develop infections that affect more than 1 million people annually [1]. Bacterial infections are caused by the presence and proliferation of microorganisms that damage host tissue. Bacterial infections are responsible for more deaths in critical care units than trauma events across the globe!

When patients have invasive procedures, research supports that bacterial contamination of the hands of hospital personnel during routine procedures is a main route for the spread of infection [2]. The purposes of this article are to identify how bacteria are classified and to review the pathophysiology of bacterial growth, bacterial transmission, nursing assessment, prevention, and management of bacterial infections.

Bacteria

Bacteria are microscopic, single-celled microorganisms that replicate by dividing [3]. Bacteria have been identified that can thrive in environments with temperatures above the boiling point and at the freezing level. Many bacteria use the human body as a source for nutrition and an environment for growth. In the human body, bacteria live on skin, in the airway, mouth, alimentary canal, and genitourinary tracts. Many bacteria grow on nonliving surfaces also, hence the need for health care providers to ascribe to meticulous aseptic techniques when providing direct patient care. Only a few bacterial types can cause disease. Bacteria generate toxins that cause cellular damage. Some bacterial infections are contagious, such as strep throat (streptococcus), whereas others, such as osteomyelitis and endocarditis, are not [4]. Common bacteria that cause infectious diseases are depicted in Table 1 [3]. Bacteria are transmitted through direct and indirect contact, airborne or droplet, and through vector transmission [3]. Examples are listed below:

- Direct contact: human bodily fluid contact, contaminated water and food sources
- Indirect contact: transmission through inanimate objects
- Airborne or droplet: talking, coughing, or currents of air
- Vector: involves insects (flies and mosquitos), also rodents (mice, rats, guinea pigs, hamsters, gerbils)

Bacterial classification

There are three ways to classify bacteria [4,5]. The information that follows helps to classify specific bacteria types.

- Shape: spherical are cocci, rod like bacteria are bacilli, and helical or spiral are spirochetes. Microscopic shape of bacteria helps to classify the specific bacteria type, thereby

* Corresponding author.
  E-mail address: lparsons@mtsu.edu (L.C. Parsons).

Table 1
Common bacteria that cause infectious disease

Bacteria/disease process	Type/ morphology	Transmission	Pathologic effects	Nursing management
Clostridium tetani (tetanus)	Gram-positive bacillus; spore-forming	Spores distributed in soil and intestinal tract of humans and animals. Infects wounds from injury.	Clinical manifestations caused by spore generation of exotoxin with affinity for CNS. S/S include neck stiffness, dysphagia, muscle rigidity.	Treated with tetanus antitoxin or immune globulins. Prevention with tetanus toxoid. May require mechanical ventilation.
Clostridium botulinum (botulism)	Gram-positive bacillus; spore-forming	Inhabits soil; frequent contaminant of fruits, vegetables, and fish. Spores are highly heat resistant.	Life-threatening paralytic illness is caused by neurotoxins. Prevents release of Ach from nerve terminals of neuromuscular junction. Damage to cranial nerves causes vision, hearing, and speech difficulties.	Treated with antitoxin from horse serum that only affects circulating toxin; has no effect on toxin bound to nerve cells. Recovery is very gradual over weeks to months.
Corynebacterium diphtheriae (diphtheria)	Gram-positive; non–spore-forming	Airborne droplets colonizing in upper respiratory system	Produces toxin resulting in epithelial cell necrosis. Inflammatory response causes production of pseudomembrane that may lead to suffocation.	Antitoxin must be administered before cell penetration by toxin. Should test for hypersensitivity to horse serum proteins before administration. Prevention is through vaccine. Penicillin may be used but is rarely effective when used alone.
Escherichia coli (coliform bacteria)	Gram-negative, non–spore-forming rods	Normal resident bacteria of intestines. May spread to urinary tract or wounds directly through fecal contamination or through the blood.	Frequent source of nosocomial infection. S/S include fever and chills. May develop shock from endotoxins. Also frequent cause of urinary tract infections.	Prevention through good handwashing and hygiene practices. Treated with cephalosporins, fluoroquinolones, or aminoglycosides. Should monitor for nephrotoxicity and ototoxicity with aminoglycosides.
Klebsiella pneumoniae	Gram-negative rod, heavily encapsulated	Found in soil, water, food, and intestinal tract.	Also associated with hospital-acquired infections. Responsible for severe respiratory tract infections in debilitated patients. S/S include productive cough and weakness.	Treated with aminoglycosides and later-generation cephalosporins. Aminoglycosides bind to ribosomes and prevent protein synthesis in bacteria. Cephalosporins interfere with cell wall synthesis.

Organism	Morphology	Characteristics	Treatment
Pseudomonas	Gram-negative rod	Common resident of skin and mucous membranes. Spreads through direct contact.	Major threat to hospitalized and debilitated patients.	Treated with aminoglycosides and later-generation cephalosporins.
Helicobacter pylori	Gram-negative spiral or straight rod	Penetrates gastric mucosa and colonizes gastric epithelium.	Produces enzyme urease that increases pH, allowing bacteria to survive in normally acidic environment. Urea in stomach is converted to ammonia, which is cytotoxic to gastric cells. Causes depletion of gastric mucus, allowing erosion of mucosa.	Treated with macrolides clarithromycin (Biaxin) and metronidazole (Flagyl). Macrolides inhibit protein synthesis, while metronidazole disrupts DNA synthesis. Alcohol should be avoided with metronidazole. Macrolides have frequent interaction with drugs.
Haemophilus influenza	Gram-negative bacillus	Occurs only in humans; more common in children than adults. Transmitted person-to-person through respiratory route.	Virulence enhanced by polysaccharide capsule that resists action of complement. Does not produce exotoxin and endotoxin does not seem to play a significant role. Results in otitis media, sinusitis, and respiratory tract infections.	Prevention is through vaccine. Drugs of choice for treatment are ampicillin or cephalosporins.
Neisseria gonorrhoeae (gonorrhea)	Gram-negative diplococcus	Transmitted through sexual contact. Primary site of infection is the cervix. Primary site in men is the urethra.	Bacteria contain pili that aid in attachment to mucosal surfaces in humans and inhibit phagocytosis. Most strains produce extracellular proteases that inactivate immunoglobulins. They also produce a cytotoxic factor that damages ciliated epithelial cells. May be asymptomatic in women but result in salpingitis, pelvic inflammatory disease, and infertility; men generally experience purulent discharge and dysuria and may experience urethral stricture.	Drug of choice is a cephalosporin, such as ceftriaxone (Rocephin). TMP/SMX (Bactrim) and ciprofloxacin (Cipro) may also be used. Ciprofloxacin inhibits DNA replication, whereas TMP/SMX prevents synthesis of proteins and nucleic acid. Patient should be instructed to avoid unprotected sexual contact.

(continued on next page)

Table 1 (*continued*)

Bacteria/disease process	Type/morphology	Transmission	Pathologic effects	Nursing management
Staphylococcus	Gram-positive cocci that grow in clusters of short chains.	Transmitted through hair follicles into the bloodstream or through the urinary or respiratory tract.	Common resident of skin. Hardy non–spore-forming bacteria that are heat stable. Anaerobes that produce enzyme catalase. Some forms produce coagulase causing clots in citrated plasma. Pathogenic staphylococcus releases several toxins, including hemolysins, leukocidin, enterotoxins, and exfoliation. They have also been implicated in toxic shock syndrome.	Humans have high resistance to staphylococcus because of development of high antibody titers. Penicillinase-resistant penicillins and cephalosporins are the drugs of choice; however, resistant strains have developed. Vancomycin (Vancocin) is the drug of choice for methicillin-resistant strains. It interferes with cell wall synthesis. In cases in which resistance has developed to vancomycin, drugs such as quinupristin and dalfopristin (Synercid) and linezolid (Zyvox) or combination therapy using vancomycin and gentamicin have been effective.
Streptococcus	Gram-positive cocci that grow in chains or as diplococci.	Transmitted through respiratory droplets or direct contact with secretions.	Group A beta-hemolytic streptococcus produces erythrogenic toxin responsible for rash in scarlet fever. Two hemolysins are produced, in addition to streptokinase, that promote lysis of human blood clots. Disease produced includes pharyngitis, otitis media, peritonsillar abscesses, meningitis, and pneumonia. Glomerulonephritis and rheumatic fever are complications that can result from streptococcal infection.	Penicillin is the drug of choice, with erythromycin used for those allergic to penicillin. Patients should be instructed in the importance of completing the entire course of prescribed antibiotics.

| *Mycobacterium tuberculosis* (tuberculosis) | Acid-fast and aerobic bacillus (caused by large amounts of lipid in cell wall) | Tubercle is transmitted through respiratory droplets from humans, cows, or birds. May also enter blood and lymph system and travel to other parts of the body. | Grows slowly and often results in self-limiting lesion. Initial lesion appears as area of nonspecific pneumonitis. The caseous lesion heals by fibrosis and calcification. This lesion can be reactivated with low host resistance. Exotoxins or endotoxins are not produced. Mycobacteria primarily affect the lungs but may also cause infection in the kidney, liver, and genitourinary tract. | Previous mycobacterial infection can be detected through a PPD skin test; however, this does not necessarily establish the presence of active infection. The drugs of choice for treatment of tuberculosis are the antitubercular agents isoniazid (INH) and rifampin (Rifadin). These drugs interfere with protein synthesis or cell wall synthesis. Streptomycin and pyrazinamide (Tebrazid) are also used; standard antibiotics are not effective against mycobacteria. Treatment usually continues for 3 to 6 months and patient compliance must be encouraged. |

Abbreviation: S/S, signs and symptoms.

From Hogan MA, Hill K. Pathophysiology: reviews and rationales. Upper Saddle River (NJ): Prentice Hall;2004;411–14. Reprinted by permission of Pearson Education, Inc., Upper Saddle River, NJ.

providing direction to pharmacologic management of the specific microorganism (Figs. 1–3).

- Color after a Gram stain has been applied; gram-positive bacteria stain purple–blue and gram-negative bacteria stain pink–red. Gram staining is a process used to establish the chemical make-up of the cell wall of bacteria. The cell wall can stain either positive or negative, depending on its chemistry. Knowing the chemical make-up makes it easier to medically manage the specific bacteria type.
- Bacterial use of oxygen; bacteria that live and grow on the presence of oxygen are called aerobes. Bacteria that tolerate low oxygen levels or are poisoned by oxygen are called anaerobes. For this reason travelers have used stabilized oxygen or aerobic oxygen to purify their drinking water when traveling to developing countries. Aerobic oxygen kills microbes, anaerobic bacteria, and viruses [6].

Gram-positive and gram-negative bacteria produce different infections; thus, different antibiotics are used to kill these bacteria [3]. Gram-positive bacteria respond better to antibiotic therapy, whereas gram-negative bacteria have a tough outer membrane that is more difficult for drugs to penetrate. If gram-negative bacteria enter the bloodstream, the lipopolysaccharides in the outer membrane therefore trigger high fever and

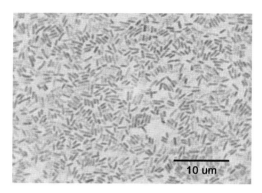

Fig. 2. Single rod (Bacillus). *From* Kaiser GE. The prokaryotic cell: bacteria. Doc Kaiser's Microbiology Homepage. http://student.ccbcmd.edu/courses/bio141/lecguide/unit1/shape/shape.html 2006. Used with permission.

life-threatening decreases in blood pressure. Bacterial lipopolysaccharides are therefore referred to as endotoxins. Gram-positive bacteria are more responsive to antibiotic therapy. Trauma and postsurgical patients have higher tendencies toward anaerobic bacterial invasion of the skin and muscle tissue, especially if tissue has a poor blood supply. Compounding medical management is that anaerobic infections frequently have a collection of purulent exudate (pus), thereby causing pain. Most anaerobic infections arise from the body's own pool of bacteria.

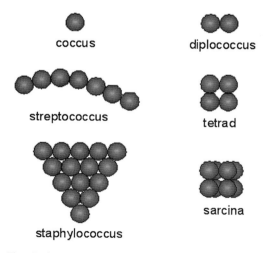

Fig. 1. Arrangements of Cocci. *From* Kaiser GE. The prokaryotic cell: bacteria. Doc Kaiser's Microbiology Homepage. http://student.ccbcmd.edu/courses/bio141/lecguide/unit1/shape/shape.html 2006. Used with permission.

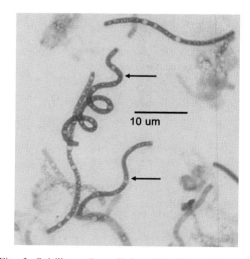

Fig. 3. Spirillum. *From* Kaiser GE. The prokaryotic cell: bacteria. Doc Kaiser's Microbiology Homepage. http://student.ccbcmd.edu/courses/bio141/lecguide/unit1/shape/shape.html 2006. Used with permission.

Pathophysiology

Bacterial proliferation depends on the body's immune system and the capacity of bacteria to oppose the body's natural defense mechanisms [3,7]. The skin and mucous membranes are the external barriers that are the body's first line of defense against infectious microorganisms [8]. The gastrointestinal, respiratory, and genitourinary tracts form a closed barrier between the visceral organ systems and the environment. Cells of innate resistance (immunity) emit a Toll-like receptor that interacts with pathogens and activates inflammation and adaptive immunity: the second and third lines of defense against infectious bacteria.

Once bacteria penetrate the skin and mucous membranes, the inflammatory process is initiated, mainly through phagocytes. Phagocytosis, frequently referred to as cell eating, occurs when neutrophils attack bacteria and destroy the microorganism. Antibiotics are often necessary to assist the immune system in killing destructive bacteria.

The transmission of infection, referred to as the chain of infection, is a series of events that occurs when the bacterial microorganism reaches a susceptible host [3]. If an individual lacks resistance to the invading bacteria, illness ensues.

Clinical manifestations

A patient may be asymptomatic when a pathogen is present for hours or years during the incubation period [3,9]. When illness presents, initial symptoms may include generalized malaise and weakness, loss of appetite, and headache. Eventually symptoms may include fever, muscle aches, diarrhea, and organ-specific manifestations, such as urinary tract infection and sore throat. Lymph node tenderness and enlargement may occur also.

Vulnerable cohorts

Children and elders are at higher risk for infectious processes [3,9]. Invasion of the major lines of defense of the integument and altered immune system functions contribute to the risk for prolonged bacterial infections. Smoking and excessive alcohol consumption interfere with the vascular system, reducing the patient's ability to kill off the invading bacteria with antibiotic therapy.

Research supports that men are at higher risks for major infections following surgery [10]. Males experiencing trauma events following injuries of moderate severity were 58% more vulnerable for developing major infections when compared with their female counterparts (Fig. 4).

Nursing assessment

Assessment includes identifying affected organ systems by the bacterial infection. The portals of entry for many bacterial infections are the respiratory tract, gastrointestinal tract, genitourinary tract, skin and mucous membranes, and the bloodstream. The assessment must include:

- Systems-specific assessment
- Temperature
- Mental status
- Pain status
- Palpation of lymph nodes

Urinary tract infection (UTI) is a common health care alteration-associated illness [9]. More than 50% of patients in intensive care units have indwelling urinary catheters, which are the primary cause of UTIs [11]. Researchers have found that urinary catheters coated with silver alloy may reduce the risk for UTIs [12,13].

Invasive devices frequently used in acute and critical care units, such as central venous pressure (CVP) lines, intubation during mechanical ventilation, and other tubes, facilitate direct access of microorganisms into the bloodstream [9]. The National Nosocomial Infection Surveillance (NNIS) reports that for every 1000 days that CVP lines are used in critical care and acute medical-surgical units, close to five infections result [13]. Technology advances may improve materials used to make catheters and other invasive tubes to reduce risk factors associated with bacterial bloodstream infections. Home health care nurses have seen insect bite (vector) infections that have caused bloodstream infections also.

Diagnostic tests

The following diagnostic and laboratory tests contribute to assessment information for critical care nurses [3]. Culture and sensitivity identify the invading microorganism, thereby facilitating the selection of the most effective antibacterial agent to kill the bacteria.

Complete blood count (CBC) to include:

- White blood count elevated to $> 10,000/mm^3$
- Neutrophil count elevated with most bacterial infections (severe bacterial infections may cause neutropenia)

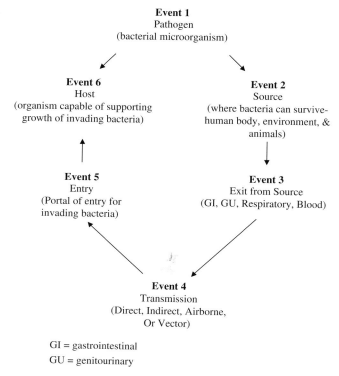

Event 1
Pathogen
(bacterial microorganism)

Event 6
Host
(organism capable of supporting
growth of invading bacteria)

Event 2
Source
(where bacteria can survive-
human body, environment, &
animals)

Event 5
Entry
(Portal of entry for
invading bacteria)

Event 3
Exit from Source
(GI, GU, Respiratory, Blood)

Event 4
Transmission
(Direct, Indirect, Airborne,
Or Vector)

GI = gastrointestinal
GU = genitourinary

Fig. 4. Chain of infection.

- Culture and sensitivity (identifies specific bacterial organism and determines most effective antibiotic to kill bacteria)
- Gram stain (allows presumptive identification of bacterial classification)

Table 2 reviews common bacterial disease examples and their disease manifestations.

Nursing management

Nurse practice in all health care settings must include strict aseptic technique. Hand washing between each procedure goes far in preventing the spread of any infection [14,15]. The bedside nurse must use strict adherence to isolation precautions to decrease the possibility of bacterial spread [16] (Box 1).

Use protective barriers when caring for patients who have bacterial infections, including disposable gowns, gloves, masks, and glasses (goggles) [17]. Teach patients to take all antibacterial medication for the prescribed duration, with a special emphasis on continuing to take medication even if symptoms of illness subside. Patients

and their visitors must be taught proper hand hygiene and to use interventions (cover mouth when coughing) that prevent the spread of infection. The critical care nurse should not assume visitors know how to prevent the spread of infection and should teach disease prevention techniques. It is helpful to have signage in prominent view for staff

Table 2
Bacterial infectious organisms

Bacteria/disease process	Common disease manifestations
Staphylococcus	Superficial skin infections, pneumonia, urinary tract infections, pneumonia, bacteremia
Streptococcus	Skin infections, pharyngitis, pneumonia
Neisseria meningitidis	Meningitis
Escherichia coli	Urinary tract infection, (frequent source for nosocomial infections)
Pseudomonas aeruginosa	Skin and mucous membrane infection, otitis, urinary tract infection

Box 1. Hand hygiene guidelines

Hand hygiene (washing hands or use of alcohol-based solution) decreases outbreaks in hospitals, reduces transmission of antimicrobial organisms (eg, MRSA), and decreases infection rates

Traditional handwashing with soap and water and use of alcohol-based solutions

When hands are visibly soiled, the nurse should wash hands with soap and water.

Gloves should be changed before and after use for individual procedures. Gloves reduce hand contamination by up to 80%.

Hand hygiene must be done after gloves have been removed. Gloves are not impervious barriers to objects with which they come in contact.

Apply alcohol-based solution to the palm of one hand, covering all surfaces of both hands and fingers.

Alcohol-based solutions reduce the number of microorganisms on the skin, have decreased skin irritation, and are fast acting.

Do not wear artificial fingernails or nail extenders, because they are associated with infectious outbreaks.

Alcohol-based solution use takes less time than traditional handwashing. This saves the critical care nurse close to 13% of their time in an 8-hour shift.

and visitors explaining special precautions and hand hygiene protocols. Patients should balance rest with care activities. The nurse must curb visitation if the patient is too fatigued and needs to sleep versus entertain visitors. It is important that the patient have a balanced diet, and fluids must be encouraged. Finally, collection of laboratory specimens is needed to identify specific bacterial microorganisms so the correct antibacterial drugs can be prescribed to kill the invading bacteria.

Summary

Acute and critical care nurses must maintain a current knowledge base for advancing science

and providing direct care for patients. When an infectious process is involved, it is the practicing nurse who must be knowledgeable in treatment and prevention modalities.

The integument is the body's first line of defense for invading bacteria. This barrier to bacteria is followed by inflammation and adaptive immunity, the second and third lines of defense against infectious bacteria. It is acute and critical care nurses, however, who should be the first line of defense in preventing the spread of infectious disease. Modern medicine and common sense interventions reviewed in this article are the patient's best defense to good health and wellness when used by nurses.

References

[1] Encyclopedia of surgery: a guide for patients and caregivers. Hospital-acquired infections. Available at: http://www.surgeryencyclopedia.com/Fi-La/Hospital-Acquired-Infections.html. Date accessed: May 15, 2006.

[2] Pittet D, Dharan S, Tiuveneau S, et al. Bacterial contamination of the hands of hospital staff during routine patient care. Arch Intern Med 1999;159:821–6.

[3] Hogan MA, Hill K. Pathophysiology: reviews and rationales. Upper Saddle River (NJ): Prentice Hall; 2004.

[4] Steckleberg J, Mayo Clinic Medical Services. Viral infections and bacterial infections: what's the difference? Available at: http://www.mayoclinic.com/health/infectious-disease/AN00652. Date accessed: May 15, 2006.

[5] Kaiser GE. The prokaryotic cell: bacteria. Sizes, shapes, and arrangements of bacteria. Doc Kaiser's Microbiology Homepage. Available at: http://student.ccbcmd.edu/courses/bio141/lecguide/unit1/shape/shape.html. Date accessed: May 15, 2006.

[6] Storehouse Foods and Botanicals. Stabilized oxygen. Available at: http://www.foodreserves.com/stabilized-oxygen.html. Date accessed: May 15, 2006.

[7] Bullock BA, Henze R. Focus on pathophysiology. Philadelphia: Lippincott; 2000 Center for Disease Control (CDC). Fact Sheet: Hand hygiene guidelines fact sheet. Available at: http://www.cdc.gov/od/oc/media/pressrel/fs021025.htm. Date accessed: May 15, 2006.

[8] McCance LM, Huether SE. Pathophysiology: the biologic basis for disease in adults and children. St. Louis (MO): Elsevier, Mosby; 2006.

[9] Ignatavicius DD, Workman ML. Medical-surgical nursing—critical thinking for collaborative care. St. Louis (MO): Elsevier, Saunders; 2006.

[10] Offner PH, Moore EE, Biffl WL. Male gender is a risk factor for major infections after surgery. Arch Surg 1999;134(9):935–40.

[11] National Nosocomial Infections Surveillance System. National Nosocomial Infections Surveillance (NNIS) system report, data summary from January 2002–June 2002. Atlanta (GA): Hospital Infection Program, National Center for Infectious Diseases, Centers for Disease Control and Prevention; 2002.

[12] Saint S, Veenstra DC, Sullivan SD, et al. The potential clinical and economical benefits of silver alloy urinary catheters in preventing urinary tract infections. Arch Intern Med 2000;160:2670–5.

[13] Saint S, Wiese J, Amory JK, et al. Are physicians aware of which of their patients have indwelling urinary catheters? Am J Med 2000;109: 476–80.

[14] Centers for Disease Control and Prevention (CDC). Guidelines for hand hygiene in health-care settings: recommendations of the Healthcare Infection Control Practices Advisory Board Committee and the HICPAC/SHEA/APIC/IDSA Hand Hygiene Task Force. MMWR Morb Mortal Wkly Rep 2002; 51(RR-16):1–44.

[15] Department of Health and Human Services, Centers for Disease Control and Prevention. National Nosocomial Infections Surveillance System (NNIS). Available at: http://www.cdc.gov/ncidod/dhqp/nnis. html. Date accessed: May 15, 2006.

[16] McGee EJ. Necrotizing fasciitis: review of pathophysiology, diagnosis, and treatment. Crit Care Nurs Q 2005;28:80–4.

[17] Doenges ME, Moorhouse MF, Geissler AC. Nursing care plans: guidelines for individualizing client care. 5th edition. Philadelphia: FA Davis; 2000.

ELSEVIER
SAUNDERS

Crit Care Nurs Clin N Am 19 (2007) 27–38

CRITICAL CARE
NURSING CLINICS
OF NORTH AMERICA

Rickettsial and Other Tick-Borne Infections

Barbara Fouts Flicek, MSN, RN, FNP

Internal Medicine of Newton County, 4181 Hospital Drive NE, Suite 404, Covington, GA 30014

Rickettsia are small pleomorphic coccobacilli that are obligate intracellular parasites. Most *Rickettsia* species exert their effect by producing a vasculitis by infecting the endothelia of capillaries, small arteries, and small veins [1,2]. Transmission from animal to human is normally through an arthropod, the most common being a tick. Tick-borne illnesses and rickettsial diseases continue to cause severe illness and death in otherwise healthy adults and children, despite the availability of low-cost, effective antimicrobial therapy. Early signs and symptoms of these illnesses often mimic a benign or nonspecific viral illness, making diagnosis difficult. This difficult diagnostic dilemma is the greatest challenge to clinicians, because antibiotic therapy is most effective in the early clinical course of these infections. This has definite implications for critical care nurses who practice in primary care settings as acute care nurse practitioners, as well as those who practice in tertiary care centers with in-patient populations.

The *Rickettsia* species of the spotted fever group is primarily transmitted through ticks, except the *Rickettsia akari*, which is transmitted through mites and causes rickettsialpox [1]. The primary vectors for the typhus group *Rickettsia* are human body lice, lice, and fleas [1]. Tick-borne diseases are the most common vector-borne *Rickettsia* in the United States [3], and worldwide are only second to msquitos in the transmission of diseases. Although certain ticks are endogenous to certain geographic locations, infectious challenges in one geographic region have the potential for transforming into more global problems. Nile disease and monkeypox are examples of diseases that can spread globally by human travelers, animal migration, or importation, as well as by vector transport from one region to another.

The concept that ticks were not pathogenic to humans was drastically modified from 1984 to 2005 with the identification of at least 11 rickettsial species or subspecies that caused tick-borne rickettsial infections around the world [4]. During the last 20 years, the recognition of multiple distinct tick-borne rickettsioses has been facilitated by advances in technology, particularly the broad use of cell cultures and the development of molecular methods from human samples and ticks [5]. This is important for early recognition of rickettsial infections. The critical care nurse is more likely to encounter ticks and tick-borne illnesses as opposed to other forms of *Rickettsia*. For this reason, the discussion in this article is limited to ticks and tick-borne illnesses.

Anatomy of a tick bite

The mechanism by which a disease is transmitted by a tick is not well understood. There is support that during a blood meal, the pathogen that is harbored in the gastrointestinal tract of the tick migrates to their salivary glands. When the tick attaches to a human there are prostaglandins released from the saliva of the tick to the host. The myriad of actions caused by these prostaglandins inhibit the human immune response. Apyrase, an enzyme in tick saliva, is thought to augment blood flow at the bite by causing vasodilation [3]. It also inhibits the formation of a clot at the site by preventing platelet aggregation. There are also other agents in tick saliva that inhibit clotting that facilitate the transmission of infectious agents to the host [6]. The clinical manifestations of many rickettsioses such as hypvolemia and edema of the skin, lungs, and brain are thought to be the result of increased vascular

E-mail address: stephen.krau@vanderbilt.edu

permeability. This is the key event that results in microvascular leakage as a systemic endothelial infection [6].

Classifications of ticks

In the event that the critical care nurse encounters a patient who has received a tick bite, or has a tick attached to his or her person, it is important to identify the type of tick and classification for proper treatment. Ticks are blood-sucking ectoparasites that act as vectors for rickettsial, spirochetal bacterial, and parasitic infections. Adult ticks of some species can reach up to 1 cm in length. Ticks have eight legs, and the front two are curved forward, similar to a crab. Ticks are members of the class Arachnida, and there are three families of ticks, two of which are known to transmit disease to humans [3,7]. The hard-bodied Ixodidae includes 13 genera. Of these 13, only Amblyomma, Dermacentor, and Ioxides transmit disease to humans in the United States. The family of soft-bodied ticks, Argasidae, contain five genera. Of these, only the Ornithodoros is known to transmit disease to humans in the United States [3]. A third family, the *Nuttalliellidae*, is represented by only a single species that is confined to southern Africa. Table 1 provides an overview of the soft tick, and the hard tick most prominently found in North America.

Disease-transmitting hard ticks

The deer tick

The deer tick (*Ixodes dammini*) is responsible for the transmission of Lyme disease and human babesiosis. This tick is found in areas such as Massachusetts, Connecticut, New Jersey, and the islands of coastal New England. This tick is more common in southern Connecticut, and has parasitized three different host animals during its 2-year life cycle. Larval and nymphal ticks have parasitized 31 different species of mammals and 49 species of birds [8]. The crucial host for adult ticks appears to be the white-tailed deer. Humans, unfortunately, may be the host during all three feeding stages of the tick. Most infections are acquired from feeding nymphs in May through early July. Birds, other mammals, and rodents may be reservoir hosts for the spirochete. A particularly important reservoir host is the white-footed mouse. These mice abide in parts of southern Connecticut where Lyme disease is prevalent in humans. Lyme disease is caused by *Borrelia burgdorferi*, and is universally present during the summer in these mice. The proliferation of deer in North America has caused the expansion of the geographic range of these illnesses.

American dog tick

The American dog tick (*Dermacentor variabilis*) derives its common name from the fact that

Table 1
Classifications of ticks

	Soft tick	Hard tick
Family	*Argasidae*	*Ixodidae*
Anatomy		
General appearance	The body is a nondescript sac-like shape, somewhat like a large raisin; the front portion of the body extends forward, above, and beyond the base of the capitulum, and is concealed when the tick is viewed from above	Hard ticks have the capitulum (where the head and mouth parts are located) exposed and easily visible from the top; unfed hard ticks are shaped like a flat seed
Body surface	No scutum on the upper side of the body, and the exoskeleton is rather leathery in texture with a distinctly roughened surface	The upper side of the body bears a distinctly sclerotized shield or scutum
Blood meal source	Prefers to feed on birds or bats and is seldom encountered	Prefers to feed on mammals; hence the many mammal names associated with ticks
Feeding habits	Usually feed for less than 1 h	Tend to attach and feed for hours to days
Disease transmission	Can occur in less than a minute	Usually occurs near the end of a meal, as the tick becomes full of blood
Local reactions	—	Pain, erythema, and nodules
Removal	Easier to remove than hard ticks	Difficult to remove

it is only found in North America and that domestic dogs are the primary host of the adult tick. The tick is attracted to the scent of animals, and is often found in wooded areas and trails where it commonly attaches to dogs and readily attacks humans. It is of medical importance because it vectors the causal organisms of Rocky Mountain spotted fever (RMSF) and tularemia, and also causes tick paralysis. It is found throughout the United States except for the area of the Rocky Mountains, and in Canada and Mexico [9]. *Dermacentor andersoni* is the vector for RMSF in the west, and are recognized by their white-gray anterodorsal ornamentation.

The U.S. Centers for Disease Control and Prevention (CDC) recognize many new rickettsial species, and therefore emerging rickettsial diseases, but clinicians will continue to focus on spotted fever in the United States.

Rocky Mountain spotted fever (Rickettsia rickettsii)

Spotted fever group rickettsiae are obligate intracellular, arthropod-borne bacteria that compromise at least thirty diverse genotypes, which include 15 distinct species currently recognized as pathogens in humans. A newly recognized cause is *Rickettsia parkeri*, a bacterium recovered from Gulf Coast ticks (*Amblyomma maculatum*).

In the United States, three species of spotted fever group are recognized agents of human disease: *Rickettsia rickettsii*, the cause of RMSF; *Rickettsia akari*, the mite-borne agent of rickettsialpox; and *Rickettsia felis,* the cause of cat-flea spotted fever group rickettsiosis [10]. Most clinicians do not consider *Rickettsia felis*, but this unusual rickettsial disease can be associated with considerable long-term fatigue and many mysterious febrile illnesses.

Methods for identifying pathogens associated with rickettsial infections are time-consuming, and can be costly. The most common method is serologic testing. A serum specimen is evaluated for IgG antibodies that react with various spotted fever group rickettsiae by use of an indirect immunofluorescence antibody assay. Histopathologic and immunohistochemical evaluation from a punch biopsy specimen can also be done. This can only be done if a bite site and eschar are present. The pathogen may also be identified by isolation in cell culture of the punch biopsy specimen. Other methods include examination of the cells by electron microscopy and molecular analyses of DNA from biopsied tissue.

Much focus has been given to the identification of ticks, geographic distribution of vectors and disease, and identification of the disease-causing pathogen. All tick-borne illnesses present with many of the same signs and symptoms, and require prompt recognition, because death can occur without proper treatment. Table 2 provides an overview of the major ticks that cause diseases in humans in North America.

Tick-borne diseases

Lyme disease

Lyme disease is the most common tick-borne illness in the United States. The disease is caused by infection of the spirochete, *Borrelia burgdoferi*, and is the most common vector-borne illness in the United States [6,11]. After a bite from an infected tick, an incubation period of several days to 1 month may elapse before the characteristic skin lesion forms. Erythema migrans forms at the site of the bite. Common sites include the axillae, groin, and waistline. The lesion of erythema migrans starts as an erythematous macule or papule with an outer border and central clearing. The border is well demarcated, warm to touch, and nontender. This rash is the single best clinical marker for Lyme disease, occurring in up to 90% of cases. The rash resolves spontaneously within several weeks if left untreated, and in days with appropriate antibiotic therapy. Most patients have some constitutional symptoms, such as myalgia, fatigue, arthalgia, or headache. Twenty percent of the patients have manifestation other than the rash [12].

Early localized Lyme disease can progress to hematogenous dissemination within the first month. End-organ effects develop within several weeks to 1 year after the primary infection in untreated patients. Lyme disease may have neurologic, cardiac, musculoskeletal, and dermatologic manifestations. Neurologic manifestation includes meningitis, cranial neuropathy, and peripheral radiculoneuropathies. Meningitis presents with fever, headache, photophobia, and meningismus. The cerebrospinal fluid typically demonstrates a mild lymphocytic pleocytosis and an increased protein level. The most common cranial neuropathy is Bell's palsy or seventh nerve palsy. Involvement of one or more of the sensory or motor nerves of the thorax or limbs in an

Table 2
Overview of major ticks the United States

Name	Common name	Diseases transmitted	Geographic location	Description	Feeding preferences
Dermacenter variabilis	American dog tick, wood tick	Rocky Mountain spotted fever, tularemia, and possibly ehrlichiosis to humans	Throughout the United States, but mostly east of the Rocky Mountains and only sparsely in the Rocky Mountain region	Unfed males and females are reddish brown and are ~3/16 inch long; females have a large silver spot behind the head; males have silver stripes	Larva and nymphs feed on small warm-blooded animals such as birds and mice; adults feed on humans and large mammals such as dogs, deer, and raccoons
Dermacentor andersoni stiles	Rocky Mountain wood tick	Rocky Mountain spotted fever and also transmits the casual organisms of Colorado tick fever and tularemia; it also causes tick paralysis	Most arid parts of North America; central British Columbia through southern Alberta into southwestern Saskatchewan, Washington, Oregon, and California, all of Montana, Idaho, Wyoming, Nevada, and Arizona, western Oklahoma to northern New Mexico, and Texas	Brown but becomes grayish in tone when engorged; females measure 1/8 inch, males measure 1/16 to 1/4 inch	Larvae and nymphs feed mainly on rodents such as chipmunks and ground squirrels; adults prefer large animal hosts such as cattle, sheep, deer, and humans

Amblyomma americanum	Lone Star tick	Can transmit Rocky Mountain spotted fever but is less likely to do so than the American dog tick; may transmit tularemia and ehrlichiosis to humans; Southern tick-associated rash illness	Found mainly in the southeastern United States west into Texas; pockets found in New Jersey, Fire Island, NY, and Prudence Island, RI	The nymph, the most common found on people, is about the size of a pin head. Adults are brown and measure 1/8 inch; the female has a white spot in the middle of her back	Larvae, nymphs, and adults will feed on a variety of warm-blooded hosts, including humans
Ixodes cokkei Packard	Groundhog tick	—	Most common in New England, but present in all areas east of the Mississippi River	—	—
Ixodes scapularis	Blacklegged tick, deer tick, seed tick	Lyme disease, *Borrelia burgdorferi*, as well as the agents of human babesiosis, *Babesia microti*, and human granulocytic ehrlichiosis	East coast of the United States; Florida westward into central Texas and Mexico; Maine westward to Minnesota and Iowa	Approximately 3 mm and dark brown to black in color; females typically have a red or orange mark behind the scutum	All three active stages will feed on a variety of hosts, including humans; adults feed primarily on deer
Rhipicephalus sanguineus	Brown dog tick, kennel tick	Rarely cause disease in humans, but cause a series of illnesses in household pets, especially dogs	Found worldwide, though more commonly in warmer climates; present throughout Florida	Reddish-brown, about 1/8 inch long; lacks any ornamentation, and has an elongated body shape	Feeds on dogs and rarely bites people

asymmetric pattern or focal weakness is how peripheral radiculoneuropathy presents, and may often be confused with spinal discogenic pain. Within 3 months of developing erythema migrans, untreated patients may develop carditis. The incidence of Lyme carditis is unknown because most patients have asymptomatic first-degree atrioventricular block. Complete heart block, cardiomyopathy, pericarditis, and myocarditis are rare, but can occur. Cardiac involvement recedes with antimicrobial treatment, but the need for temporary pacemaker placement has occurred. Roughly half of untreated patients develop migratory arthralgias, myalgias, tendonitis, bursitis, or bone pain. Unusual manifestations include optic neuritis, hepatitis, myositis, and pneumonitis.

The diagnosis of Lyme disease should be based primarily on the presence of characteristic clinical findings, exposure to an endemic area, and response to appropriate antibiotic therapy [13]. The clinical presentation of erythema migrans is so distinctive that any patient presenting with this rash requires treatment.

Routinely available diagnostic testing determines whether there has been an immune response to the spirochete, using an ELISA to detect immunoglobulin M (IgM) and IgG antibodies to *B burgdorferi*. In patients infected with Lyme disease it takes several weeks before an IgM response can be detected. This may not occur after early antibiotic use. The CDC suggest a two-step Lyme diagnostic test strategy in which positive or equivocal ELISA studies are confirmed by Western blot testing for Lyme-specific IgM and IgG bands [12].

Rocky Mountain spotted fever

R rickettsii is the organism responsible for RMSF [3]. Howard Ricketts [6] identified the causative agent in the early 1900s. The name RMSF was coined to describe a disease that was first observed in the Bitter Root Valley of western Montana, but the disease occurs in many areas of the United States. This infection is most commonly now seen east of the Mississippi River, especially in the southeastern United States. Four states (North Carolina, Oklahoma, Tennessee, and South Carolina) account for 48% of reported illness [8].

Most cases of RMSF occur in the late spring or summer, April 1 through September 30, the period when ticks are most active. The common dog tick, *D variabilis*, transmits most cases of RMSF in the eastern United States, and the Rocky Mountain wood tick, *D andersoni*, in the West. Ticks are often brought into close contact with people via pet dogs or cats. Rocky Mountain spotted fever is caused by *R rickettsii* released from infected tick salivary glands during the 6 to 10 hours they are attached to the human host.

Children 5 to 9 years of age and young adults are most commonly infected. It is assumed that this age group is affected because of increased outdoor exposure. Initial symptoms are often mistakenly dismissed as a routine summertime viral illness with fever, severe headache, myalgia, arthralgia, and vomiting [3]. Symptoms may occur within 3 to 21 days after the bite and start abruptly. The average incubation period is 7 days. Other symptoms include nausea and vomiting.

Rash is the major diagnostic sign, occurring in 83% to 90% of infected patients [3]. The rash typically appears 3 to 5 days after the initial onset of symptoms. The characteristic maculopapular rash first erupts on the wrists and ankles. The rash involves the palms and soles, and then spreads toward the trunk, becoming more generalized. The rash is discrete, blanches with pressure, and becomes petechial [3]. Involvement of the palm and soles has been considered a standard presentation of RMSF, but it does not occur in all patients. The rash is difficult to see in African Americans, which may explain the higher fatality rate for African Americans (16%) compared with Whites (3%) [8]. A high index of suspicion is necessary in dark-skinned populations.

Rickettsia sp infect the endothelium and vessel wall, not the cerebral tissue. RMSF is a rickettsial infection primarily of endothelial cells that normally have a potent anticoagulant function. As a result of endothelial cell infection and injury, the hemostatic system shows changes that vary widely from a minor reduction in the platelet count (frequently) to severe coagulopathies, such as deep vein thrombosis and disseminated intravascular coagulation (rarely). After the tick bites, organisms disseminate via the blood stream and multiply in vascular endothelial cells, resulting in multisystem manifestations. The effects of disseminated infection of endothelial cells include increased vascular permeability, edema, hypovolemia, hypotension, prerenal azotemia, and in life-threatening cases, pulmonary edema, shock, acute tubular necrosis, and meningoencephalitis [8]. Myocarditis is a leading cause of death. Central nervous system vasculitis is also common, and manifests itself as pneumonitis and coma.

Initial lab tests often reveal a normal or slightly depressed white blood cell (WBC) count, thrombocytopenia, hyponatremia, and elevated liver transaminases. Lumbar punctures performed for the evaluation of fever and headache reveal normal cerebrospinal fluid or a predominance monocytes and an increased WBC count [14].

The prognosis in RMSF is mainly related to the timeliness of antibiotic administration. The likelihood of death is heightened if the clinician waits for the characteristic rash or laboratory confirmation of infection. The challenge, therefore, is to recognize clinical and epidemiologic features to prompt early diagnosis. Differential diagnoses includes illnesses such as measles, rubella, gastroenteritis, disseminated gonococcal disease, upper respiratory infection, typhoid, syphilis, thrombocytopenia purpura, and adverse drug reactions. A warm-weather illness in a previously healthy patient with potential tick exposure, who is ill with fever and possible rash, should prompt the consideration of RMSF as a diagnosis.

The clinical diagnosis, which is difficult, is rarely assisted by laboratory findings because antibodies are usually detected only in convalescence, and immunohistologic methods for detection of rickettsiae are unavailable in most clinics. Definitive diagnosis can be made by culture of *R rickettsii* from blood. Only about 60% of patients with RMSF recall a tick bite [15,16].

Doxycycline is the treatment of choice except for pregnant women [3]. Tetracycline, chloramphenicol, or a fluoroquinolone are also effective. Standard therapy requires administration of doxycycline 100 mg twice a day or chloramphenical (50 to 75 mg/kg per day) for 7 days. Most broad-spectrum antibiotics, including penicillins, cephalosporins, and sulfa-containing antimicrobials, are ineffective treatments for RMSF. Doxycycline is the preferred agent for children, especially those younger than 9 years of age, because of its documented effectiveness, broader margin of safety, convenient dosing schedule, and low risk of adverse effects. Doxycycline may be administered with minimal risk of dental staining.

It has been suggested that any patient in an endemic geographic area during summer months who has fever, myalgia, and headache, receive a therapeutic trial of tetracycline, due to the fact there is no reliable early diagnostic test. Although tetracyclines are not usually given to children because of staining of dental enamel, a single course is unlikely to damage teeth. Therefore, tetracycline should not be withheld in children suspected of having RMSF.

Ehrlichioses

Only recently has human infection by the genus *Ehrlichia* been known in the United States. Ehrlichiae have been known for a long time as veterinary pathogens. Infection with this rickettsial agent produces an illness much like RMSF, but has no rash. The ticks that transmit these intracellular pathogens belong to the Ixodidae family. Ehrlichioses is transmitted during warm weather months and *Amblyomma americanum,* the Lone Star tick, a vector of human ehrlichliosis, attaches mainly to the lower extremities, buttocks, and groin. There have been three ehrlichi that have been reported as being pathogenic for humans. The first human case of monocytic ehrlichiosis was described in 1986, and was assumed to be due to *Ehrlichia canis*, the agent of canine ehrlichiosis. The actual agent, *Ehrlichia chaffeenis*, was isolated in 1991 in the United States [13]. Human monocytotrophic ehrlichiosis (HME) occurs most commonly in the southeastern and southcentral portion of the United States.

Most patients with HME do not have symptoms, or have only mild symptoms, and do not seek medical attention. The patients who do seek medical attention have become acutely and severely ill. Almost one half of these patients require hospitalization for fever, headache, rigors, and myalgias. Other symptoms include nausea, vomiting, and abdominal pain. All symptoms occur usually within 7 days after a tick bite. A maculopapular rash, sometimes with petechial features, may occur. Laboratory hallmarks of HME include leukopenia, thrombocytopenia, and elevations in liver transaminases. Patients who are severely ill require admission to the intensive care unit due to multiorgan system failure. Death occurs in 3% of patients, especially among the immunosuppressed [12].

Diagnosis may be made with a peripheral blood smear. Examination reveals morulae within monocytes or lymphocytes. Morulae are mulberry-like clusters of bacteria. The most sensitive laboratory test is polymerase chain reaction (PCR) detection of the organisms in blood. Paired acute/convalescent serologies can confirm diagnosis retrospectively. However, as with RMSF, clinical suspicion of ehrlichial infection is necessary, because delay of treatment increases the likelihood of complications or death.

Doxycycline (100 mg twice daily) is the treatment of choice. Symptoms may improve or resolve within 24 to 48 hours after initiation of Doxycycline, but treatment should be for a minimum course of 5 to 7 days. Chloramphenicol (Chloromycetin) and rifampin (Rifadin) are alternative treatments and recommended for 2 weeks [3]. Severe illness may take weeks to resolve, even with appropriate antibiotic therapy.

The bacterium, *Anaplasma phagocytophila*, is responsible for causing human granulocytic ehrlichiosis (HGE). This bacterium is transmitted mostly by *Ixodes persculatus*-complex ticks; therefore, it has much of the same distribution as Lyme disease. HGE produces subclinical disease in many cases, much like HME. Common symptoms include fever, headache, and myalgias, similar to HME. Leukopenia, thrombocytopenia, and liver function abnormalities are common, although neutropenia specifically distinguishes HGE from HME. Morulae are identified within the granulocytes in up to 80% of the patients. The treatment regimen is identical to that for HME.

Other diseases

Babesiosis

Babesiosis is a protozoal tick-borne infection, occurring in geographic regions of similar distribution to Lyme disease. The primary vector is *Ixodes scapularis*, and is found in coastal New England and mid-Atlantic regions.

Illness typically begins 1 to 6 weeks after a tick bite with malaise, fever, headache, myalgia, and loss of appetite. Babesia invades erythrocytes, and causes an illness sometimes confused with malaria. Symptoms include rigors, hepatosplenomegaly. hemolytic anemia, pancytopenia, and high fevers to 40°C. Patients infected with babesia are adults, and tend to be older than 50 years of age. The illness may progress to adult respiratory distress syndrome.

Diagnosis is established by a peripheral blood smear and the observation of small, oval-ring forms of the parasite in 1% to 10% of erythrocytes. This sometimes causes confusion with ring forms of falciparum malaria [12].

Many patients infected with babesia recover without treatment. The immunocompromised patient, or the patient that has undergone a splenectomy, are at the greatest risk of severe disease.

Patients with severe illness and profound anemia may require blood transfusions. Treatment with oral clindamycin (600 mg) and quinine (650 mg) every 8 hours for 7 to 10 days has proved most efficacious.

Relapsing fever

Relapsing fever is an arthropod-borne spirochetal disease that is caused by numerous *Borrelia* species. Endemic relapsing fever is transmitted by hard ticks *Borrelia hermsii* and *Borelia duttonii*, and the soft tick genus *Ornithodoros* in North America.

Episodes of symptoms and fever alternate with an afebrile phase for 1 week or longer before returning. The symptoms are usually milder than the initial phase. The return of fever correlates with the presence of spirochetes in the blood. Most patients have a total of two to four relapses on average.

The symptoms of relapsing fever include high fever, shaking chills, headache, myalgia, arthralgia, lethargy, and sometimes photophobia. Rarely, hepatosplenomegaly, lymphadenopathy, and a petechial rash can occur. Other rare symptoms include neurologic abnormalities such as facial palsy, myelitis, and radiculopathy.

Diagnosis is made by observation of the spirochete in a peripheral blood smear. Serology tests may be falsely positive for Lyme disease, even though the blood rarely contains *Borrelia* during afebrile periods.

Treatment is tetracycline (500 mg) four times a day or doxycycline (100 mg) twice a day for 10 days. The first dose of doxycycline should be 200 mg. Patients presenting with severe illness and neurologic disease require admission to the hospital and treatment with parental antibiotics. Those antibiotics are typically ceftriaxone (2 g intravenously every day) or penicillin G (4 mU intravenously every 4 hours), for a minimum of 14 days.

Colorado tick fever

Colorado tick fever is a tick-borne viral infection caused by the bite of the wood tick *D andersoni* and the transmission of Coltivirus. This viral infection is self-limited, usually necessitating only supportive care. The main symptom is a remitting fever of 2-day intervals that lasts for about 2 weeks. Some patients describe abdominal complaints, and leukopenia is frequently observed. Colorado tick fever is often confused with RMSF, ehrlichiosis, or relapsing fever so an empiric prescription of doxycycline is advised until confirmative diagnosis. Diagnosis may be made by viral culture or viral antigen detection assays.

Tick paralysis

Another tick-borne illness to be aware of is tick paralysis. Prolonged attachment (5–7 days) of certain species of ticks may result in paralysis of the host. This disease is cause by neurotoxic substances produce by the salivary glands of attached engorged ticks. The tick is usually female. Tick paralysis is now known to occur in may countries worldwide. The most common source for this disease in the United States is a tick bite from *D andersonii and D variabilis*. Tick paralysis may occur in all age groups, but children are more commonly affected. Symptoms start with weakness of the lower extremities, ascending to the trunk musculature, upper extremities, and the head within hours or days. The patient may present with ataxia and even respiratory distress.

Tularemia

Tularemia has become more rare, but it can occur in rural populations, especially hunters. This infection is caused by the gram-negative bacterium, *Francisella tularensis*. The dog tick, *D variabilis*, and the Lone Star tick, *A americanum* are the vectors for the disease in the United States. The disease typically presents with skin involvement. The skin tends to ulcerate and form an eschar. Regional lymph nodes that drain the ulcer may become suppurative and enlarged. Most patients identify generalized symptoms such as fever, chills, headache, malaise, anorexia, fatigue, cough, myalgias, vomiting, sore throat, chest discomfort, abdominal pain, and diarrhea [3]. Depending on the type, there could be early signs of photophobia and excessive lacrimation. If the tularemia is pneumatic type, acute respiratory distress may be present. In these cases, a chest radiograph may reveal infiltrates, hilar adenopathy, and/or pleural effusions [17,18].

Diagnosis of tularemia is usually based on history and physical examination. Routine lab tests are typically nonspecific, although WBC count and estimated sedimentation rate may be normal or slightly elevated [3]. The organism can be cultured, but if done, it must be done with caution due to the risk of transmission to laboratory personnel. It takes 2 weeks for serology to confirm the diagnosis [7,18].

Unless meningitis is present, Streptomycin is the drug of choice. Alternative treatments include gentamicin, tetracycline, chloramphenicol, and fluroquinolones. Pharmacologic treatment is recommended for 7 to 14 days [18].

Q fever begins suddenly, with high fever, severe headache, malaise, and myalgia, as with other tick-borne illnesses. Acute cases also include nausea, vomiting, diarrhea, abdominal pain, and chest pain. Only about one-half of all patients infected with *C burnetii*, the causative agent, show signs of clinical illness. The other one-half that develop symptoms may progress to sore throat, chills, sweats, non-productive cough, pneumonia, and confusion. Most patients return to good health without any treatment. Only 1%–2% of patients with Q fever die of the disease [19]. Q fever may become chronic, lasting more than six months. Serious complications of chronic Q fever include hepatitis and endocarditis. Most patients that develop endocarditis have pre-existing valvular heart disease, or history of a vascular graft. Patients with chronic kidney disease, cancer, or a transplantrecipient are at risk for developing chronic Q fever. As many as 65% of patients with chronic Q fever may die of the disease [19].

A diagnosis is made by serologic testing to detect the presence of antibodies to *Coxiella burnetii* antigens, usually by immunofluorescence assay. Doxycycline is the treatment of choice for acute Q fever: 100 mg twice daily of doxycycline is the prescribed therapy, but the length of therapy should be extended to 14 to 21 days. Antibiotic therapy is most effective when initiated within the first 3 days of illness [19].

Global rickettsial infections

Discussion of diseases related to *Rickettsia* infections and tick-borne illnesses has been limited to those primarily seen in North America. Due to the current globalization and travel, boundaries are blurred, and there are illnesses indigenous to other countries. This has made the management of rickettsials much more challenging. A table of some of these *Rickettsia*-related illnesses with a brief description are presented in Table 3 [20–28].

Summary

Tick bites are best prevented by people avoiding tick-infested areas. When this is not possible, tick bites may be prevented by the wearing of long trousers that are tucked into boots. The best method to avoid tick bites is twofold: application of a topical deet (*N,N*-diethyl-*m*-toluamide) repellent to exposed skin, and treatment of clothing

Table 3
Rickettsial infections worldwide

Disease	Rickettsia	Endemic area	Brief description	Mortality
Mediterranean spotted fever	R conorii ssp conorii	Mediterranean region, including northern Africa and southern Europe	Asymptomatic incubation of 6 days followed by high fever, flulike symptoms, and black eschar at bite; a generalized maculopapular rash may develop; patients usually recover in 10 days, except in severe forms where multiorgan involvement may occur [20]	Estimated rate of ∼ 2.5% [21,22]
Israeli spotted fever	R conorii ssp israelensis	Primarily in Israel	Typical spotted fever, but eschar at bite site usually absent; usually a pink papule at site of bite [23]; splenomegaly and hepatomegaly seen in about 30% to 35% of cases [3]	Known to be fatal by causing multiorgan failure and/or septic shock
Siberian tick typhus, or North Asian tick typhus	R sibirica ssp sibirica	Many cases documented in the former Soviet Union, with 80% in western Siberia; also Northern China, where it is known as Asian tick typhus	Incubation period is 4 to 7 days following the bite; high fever associated with eschar at bite that is often accompanied by lymphadenopathy; symptoms include severe headache, myalagia, and digestive disturbances [3]	Although central nervous system involvement may occur, overall this disease is mild and is rarely associated with severe complications [3]
Queensland tick typhus	R australis	Entire eastern coast of Australia	Characterized by a sudden onset of fever, headache, and myalgia; subsequent maculopapular to vesicular rash within 10 days; inoculation eschar identifed in 65% [3]	To date, only two cases of mortality related to this disease are known [24,25]
Japanese or Oriental spotted fever	R japonica	Along the coast of southwestern and central Japan	High-risk areas include bamboo plantations and areas; abrupt onset of fever, headache, and chills; macular rash appears in 2 to 3 days over the entire body, including palms and soles; rash becomes petschial and disappears; in severe cases, disseminated intravascular coagulopathy, multiorgan failure, and acute respiratory distress syndrome have been reported [26,27]	Only one fatality has been reported to date [28]
African tick bite fever	R africae	Mainly South Africa (80%), although cases have been reported from western, central, and eastern Africa [3]	Fever is typically mild; however, multiple inoculation eschars are common, which distinguishes African tick bite fever from other spotted fever rickettsioses; vesicular rash can be seen is often accompanied by enlarged lymph nodes draining the area of the eschar [3]	No severe manifestations or deaths have been reported to date [3]

with permethrin. This system is currently used by the US Army to protect soldiers. Ticks can crawl underneath clothing and bite untreated portions of the body; therefore, treating clothing is imperative. Permethrin is nontoxic to humans, and can be used in any age group. Permethrin is commercially available.

Checking clothing regularly while in tick-infested areas is highly recommended to back up the few hours of protection provided by the insect repellents. It is also recommended that the entire body be carefully screened for ticks and other parasites by campers and hunters while they are staying in and after leaving infested areas. Any tick found should be removed immediately [19].

Removing ticks may not be easy. It is best to use blunt, rounded forceps, and a magnifying glass to remove ticks, especially when immature ticks are found. The forceps are used to grasp the mouthparts of the tick as close as possible to the skin, and then the tick is pulled upward, perpendicular to the skin, with a continuous and steady action. Usually any mouth parts of the tick retained in the skin are eliminated uneventfully by the body. Other methods of removing ticks, such as using fingers, lighted cigarettes, petroleum jelly, or suntan oil, should be avoided. Killing the tick in situ may increase the risk of regurgitation by the tick and the transmission of infectious agents [19].

Most tick bites are uncomplicated, and result only in benign cutaneous inflammatory reactions that may be pruritic for a few days. As a result of mouthparts being retained at the feeding site, a granuloma may rarely develop. There are no data to indicate that antimicrobial prophylaxsis is beneficial to the tick-bitten patient to prevent disease. It must be kept in mind that the risk of transmission of disease increases with the duration of attachment and generally requires greater than 24 to 48 hours. The degree of tick engorgement or the time since tick exposure and discovery of the tick may be used to establish the likely duration of attachment and the risk of disease transmission [13].

Reducing and controlling tick populations is difficult. Habitat modifications, including vegetation management by cutting, burning, and herbicide treatment, and drainage of wet areas are one strategy for tick control, but their effects are often short-lived, and they can cause severe ecologic damage [13]. Chemicals used to control ticks may cause environmental contamination, and therefore, toxicity for humans and animals.

Biologic control methods for ticks include the promotion of natural predators. Natural predators of ticks are beetles, spiders, and ants, and parasites such as insects, mites, and nematodes. Tick control is best based on the concept of integrated pest management, in which different control methods are adapted to one area or against one tick species with due consideration to their environmental effects [13].

Tick-borne diseases are increasing in prevalence. Perhaps it is because people are undertaking more outdoor activities, which result in contact with ticks and their pathogens. Clinicians should be aware of the clinical sign of tick-transmitted diseases, because morbidity and mortality as a result of these diseases increases substantially if there are delays in diagnosis and treatment. Tick-borne illnesses occur in distinctive geographic areas. The reporting of these illnesses and diseases to the health department enables the gathering of information and statistics. The public should be informed about the risks of disease in tick-infested areas and the means of preventing infections. The most common diseases are caused by *Rickettsia, Borrelia,* and *Ehrichia,* but with continued study, new pathogens and diseases will continue to emerge.

References

[1] Bleck TP. Central nervous system snvolvement in rickettsial diseases. Central Nervous System Infections 1999;17(4):801–12.

[2] Anderson B, Friedman H, Bendinelli M. Rickettsial infection and immunity. New York: Plenum Press; 1997.

[3] Gayle A, Ringdahl E. Tick-borne diseases. Am Fam Physician 2001;64(3):461–6.

[4] Parola P, Paddock CD, Raoult D. Tick-borne rickettsioses around the world: emerging diseases challenging old concepts. Clin Microbiol Rev 2005;18(4): 719–56.

[5] Raoult D. A new tick-borne rickettsiosis in the USA. Clin Infect Dis 2004;38:812–3.

[6] Walker DH. Targeting rickettsia. N Engl J Med 2006;354(13):1418–20.

[7] Spach DH, Liles WC, Campbell GL, et al. Tick-borne illnesses in the United States. N Engl J Med 1993;19:237–69.

[8] Habif TP. A color guide to diagnosis and therapy clinical dermatology. 4th edition. St. Louis: Mosby; 2003. 516–24.

[9] Discover life website. Updated 2006. Available at: http://pick5.pick.uga.edu/mp/20q?search= Dermacentor+variabilis. Accessed October 1, 2006.

[10] Paddock CD, Sumner JW, Comer JA, et al. Rickettsia parkeri: a newly recognized cause of spotted fever

rickettsiosis in the United States. Clin Infect Dis 2004;38:805–11.

[11] Taege AJ. Tick trouble: overview of tick-borne diseases. Cleve Clin J Med 2000;67:241, 245–9.

[12] Baker LR, Burton JR, Zieve PD, et al. Principles of ambulatory medicine. 6th edition. Philadelphia: Lippincott, Williams, and Wilkins; 2003. p. 498–507.

[13] Masur H. New organisms, new drugs, new tests, new guidelines: what do you really need to know? Available at: http://www.medscape.com/viewarticle/463990. Accessed October 1, 2006.

[14] Thorner AR, Walker DH, Petri WA Jr. Rocky Mountain spotted fever. Clin Infect Dis 1998;27:1353–60.

[15] Masters EJ, Olson GS, Weiner SJ, et al. Rocky Mountain spotted fever—a physcian's dilemma. Arch Intern Med 2003;163:769–74.

[16] Sexton DJ, Kaye KS. Rocky Mountain spotted fever. Med Clin North Am 2002;86:351–60.

[17] Cross JT, Penn RL. *Francisella tularensis* (tularemia). In: Mandell GL, Douglas RG, Bennett JE, et al, editors. Mandell, Douglas and Bennett's principles and practice of infectious diseases. 5th edition. Philadelphia: Churchill Livingstone; 2000. p. 2393–402.

[18] Cox SK, Everett ED. Tularemia, an analysis of 25 cases. Mo Med 1981;78:70–4.

[19] Center for Disease Control and Prevention. Viral and rickettsial zoonoses branch. Available at: http://www.cdc.gov/ncidod/dvrd/qfever/index.htm. Accessed October 12, 2006.

[20] Raoult DH, Gallais A, Ottomani JP, et al. Malignant form of mediterranean boutonneuse fever. 6 cases. Presse Med 1983;12:2375–8.

[21] Amaro M, Bacelar F, Franca A. Report of eight cases of fatal and severe Mediterranean spotted fever in Portugal. Ann N Y Acad Sci 2003;990:331–43.

[22] Bacellar F, Sousa R, Santos A, et al. Boutonneuse fever in Portugal: 1995–2000. Data of a state laboratory. Eur J Epidemiol 2003;18:275–7.

[23] Gross EM, Yagupsky P. Israeli rickettsial spotted fever in children. A review of 54 cases. Acta Trop 1987; 44:91–6.

[24] Graves S, Stenos J. Rickettsioses in Australia. In: Raoult D, Brouqui P, editors. Rickettsiae and rickettsial diseases at the turn of the third millennium. Paris: Elsevier; 1999. p. 244–6.

[25] Sexton DJ, Dwyer B. Fatal Queensland tick typhus. J Infect Dis 1990;162:779–80.

[26] Araki M, Takatsuka K, Kawamura J, et al. Japanese spotted fever involving the central nervous system: two case reports and a literature review. J Clin Microbiol 2002;40:3874–6.

[27] Kodama K, Senba T, Yamauchi H, et al. A patient with Japanese spotted fever complicated by meningoencephalitis. Kansenshogaku Zasshi 2001;75: 812–4.

[28] Kodama K, Senba T, Yamauchi H, et al. Fulminant Japanese spotted fever definitely diagnosed by the polymerase chain reaction method. J Infect Chemother 2002;8:266–8.

ELSEVIER
SAUNDERS

Crit Care Nurs Clin N Am 19 (2007) 39–42

CRITICAL CARE
NURSING CLINICS
OF NORTH AMERICA

Spirochete Infections: Lyme Disease and Southern Tick-Associated Rash Illness

Maria Overstreet, MSN, RN, CCNS

Vanderbilt University, School of Nursing, 303 Godchaux Hall, 461 21st Avenue South, Nashville, TN 37241, USA

In the United States 23,305 people are reported as having contracted Lyme disease during 2005 [1]. This is an increase of 3501 reported cases over a 1-year period. The initial diagnosis of Lyme disease occurred following an outbreak of arthragilias in a group of pediatric patients in 1977 in and around Lyme, Connecticut. Today, Lyme disease remains a public health concern in many parts of the United States. Ninety-seven percent of the cases in 2005 were reported from the following 13 states: New York, Pennsylvania, New Jersey, Massachusetts, Connecticut, Wisconsin, Maryland, Minnesota, Delaware, Virginia, New Hampshire, Maine, and Illinois [1].

It is important for the critical care nurse to recognize the etiology, symptoms and stages, pathophysiology, diagnosis, treatment, and prevention of Lyme disease, because some of the symptoms can have devastating effects on the heart and meninges. Acute care nurse practitioners, who might see patients exposed to these pathogens, should be aware that in some cases Lyme disease may be a comorbidity, not the primary reason a patient is admitted to an ICU. A cluster of similar symptoms called "Southern tick-associated rash illness" (STARI) results in a rash similar to that associated with Lyme disease.

Etiology of Lyme disease

Lyme disease is a vector-borne disease. It is a bacterial infection caused by a corkscrew-shaped spirochete, *Borrelia burgdorferi*. This bacterium is transmitted to humans by the Black-legged tick (*Ixodes scapularis*) found primarily in

the northeastern and north-central United States. Because there are typical times during the life cycle of this tick during which the probability of infectious bacterium pathogen transference is higher, it is important to consider the life cycle of the tick. The tick life cycle involves three stages: larva, nymph, and adult. During any of these stages the tick can become infected with the bacterium and thus can transmit the bacterium to humans. Approximately 90% of the cases contracted are transmitted during to the nymph stage of the tick life cycle [2,3]. The nymph's virulence results primarily from the length of time the host (human) allows the tick to remain attached. A nymph is approximately 2 mm in diameter; therefore, a person may not be aware of the tick's attachment, and the tick may be allowed to feed for a longer period (more than 48 hours). This prolonged attachment allows time for the bacterium to move from tick to human [2,4].

Symptoms and stages of Lyme disease

Typically, symptoms of Lyme disease present in one of three stages. The patient may experience some or all of the symptoms in each stage and may fluctuate in and out of each stage. Stage one usually occurs a few days to 1 month following a tick bite and is termed "early localized disease." The hallmark symptom is erythema migrans, a "bull's eye" rash. Nonspecific complaints resemble a viral syndrome, including malaise, fatigue, headache, myalgia, arthralgias, or generalized lymphadenopathy [2]. During the period from 1992 through 2004, of the patients reported to have Lyme disease 68% had erythema migrans, 33% had arthritis, and 1% experienced the severe symptoms of meningitis and heart block [5].

E-mail address: maria.overstreet@vanderbilt.edu

0899-5885/07/$ - see front matter © 2007 Elsevier Inc. All rights reserved.
doi:10.1016/j.ccell.2006.10.003

Stage two, early disseminated disease, can occur days to 10 months after a tick bite. At this time symptoms can include those listed for stage one along with multiple organ involvement including atrioventricular block, pericarditis, meningeal irritation, and meningitis. Additional symptoms may include palpitations, syncope, dyspnea, stiff neck, photophobia, poor memory, difficulty concentrating, paresthesia and persistent malaise, fatigue, fever, chills, and nausea.

Stage three, late persistent disease, sometimes referred to as "chronic Lyme disease," may occur months to years following a single tick bite. This patient may present with musculoskeletal and neurologic symptoms such as joint swelling, stiffness, and pain along with myalgia, fatigue, ataxia, mood changes, sleep disturbances, and personality changes.

Proposed pathophysiology of Lyme disease

It is postulated the immune system plays an integral role in the development of the various stages of Lyme disease. The body's inability to mount a sufficient immune response may be responsible for the severity of the initial or late stages of this disease.

Tick saliva also may play a role in the survival of the bacterium [6]. Within the saliva a protein may suppress the local immunoreactivity allowing the bacterium to enter a person and spread more quickly. It also is postulated that specific binding properties may allow the bacterium to disseminate more quickly to certain target tissues such as the central nervous system [6]. Still others postulate that problems may exist in the regulation of the trafficking and activation of the inflammatory cells. Sigal [6] suggests that the "immunopathogenesis of Lyme disease [may] possibly involve the following components: [i]mmunomodulation of host cells by Borrelia components, an increase in the pathogenicity of the organism by the cytokine-rich local environment, induction of arthritis by a host reaction to Borrelia antigens, and possible autoimmune reactions during the course of infection."

Coinfection also is thought to influence to the host's defense mechanisms adversely [7]. Researchers from the National Institute of Allergy and Infectious Disease have demonstrated that mice coinfected with human granulocytic ehrlichiosis suffered increased severity of Lyme disease [7]. Human granulocytic ehrlichiosis and babesiosis are found as coinfectious agents in patients who have Lyme disease [8–10].

Diagnosis of Lyme disease

A thorough patient history is one of the most important elements used in the diagnosis of Lyme disease. The patient's report of symptoms and the occurrence of and exposure to ticks in endemic areas may be the only clues to the cause of the patient's current symptoms. Diagnosis of infection remains controversial; some researchers maintain that a diagnosis of Lyme disease can be made on clinical grounds with serologies considered solely in a supportive role [11]. Blood tests may confirm Lyme disease, but a negative blood test accompanied with positive symptomology typically is considered as positive for Lyme disease. Blood tests for Lyme disease measure the body's production of antibodies to *Borrelia burgdorferi*. These tests are not able to detect acute infection until the body has been able to produce measurable amounts of antibodies, sometimes not until 2 to 8 weeks after the bite. Prevue *B. burgdorferei* (Inverness Medical Professional Diagnostics), a rapid test, can give results in 1 hour. The C6 Lyme peptide ELISA is a sensitive and specific test [12]. If the ELISA test is positive, it is customary to confirm the result by using a Western blot assay. These results take time, and treatment should be initiated with a positive patient history and symptoms without waiting for test results [11].

Treatment of Lyme disease

Lyme disease can be treated effectively with antibiotic therapy, but routine prophylactic use of antimicrobials is not recommended [8]. Some experts recommend antibiotic therapy only if certain symptoms appear or if specific epidemiologic information is available (eg, the accurate determination of the species of tick and degree of engorgement). Typically, these data are not routinely available. The most common drug of choice is doxycycline. Doxycycline, 100 mg taken orally twice daily for 14 to 21 days, is typical treatment of both stage one and two Lyme disease [8,13]. Cefuroxime axetil or erythromycin can be used (particularly in pregnant women) if the patient is allergic to penicillin or cannot take tetracyclines [13]. Treatment for third-stage or chronic Lyme disease may involve vigorous intravenous antibiotic therapy.

Ticks must be removed promptly to reduce the length of exposure. Patients admitted to the critical care unit with symptoms mimicking Lyme disease must be inspected thoroughly for ticks. Ticks should be removed with precision, using a slow, gentle, pulling motion with disposable tweezers placed as close as possible to the tick's attachment to the skin. After the tick removal, the skin should be cleaned to remove any bacteria at the site of attachment. Do not touch the tick, because the bacteria can be transmitted to the nurse. Good hand-washing practices must be employed. Make special note of where the tick was attached and any signs of a rash at the site of attachment. A rash can appear up to 1 month following removal; therefore, follow-up with a primary health care provider is encouraged.

Prevention of Lyme disease

Preventative measures and early recognition of symptoms are keys in inhibiting the occurrence of later stages of Lyme disease. Patients should be taught how to avoid future tick exposure using personal and environmental means of prevention. Avoidance of tick-infested areas, such as wooded areas or leaf piles, is paramount. Patients who enjoy hiking should stay near the center of paths, routinely perform thorough, naked-body inspection, and remove ticks promptly. Tick repellents should be applied while the hiker is in the wooded areas but should be washed off immediately afterwards. Washing with a cloth provides enough gentle friction to disturb the tick's connection to skin if performed immediately after attachment.

Patients who have Lyme disease in critical care

Lyme disease left untreated may result in varying degrees of permanent damage:

Musculoskeletal system: joints with pain and swelling progressing to arthritis

Central nervous system: facial nerve paralysis, visual disturbances, meningitis, encephalitis, memory loss, difficulty concentrating, mood changes, personality changes, and altered sleeping habits

Cardiac system: irregularities of heart rhythm, carditis, and transient atrioventricular blocks of varying degree

Chances of recovery are based on the early recognition of symptoms and treatment. Treatment of chronic Lyme disease may elicit full recovery, or the patient may be left with any or all of the symptoms listed previously.

A case study

Joseph is a 45-year-old white man admitted from the emergency department to the critical care unit with a diagnosis of fever of unknown origin. His temperature on arrival is 101.5°F. He complains of severe fatigue, headache, and muscle and joint pain. He arrives with his spouse of 20 years, who is knowledgeable and willing to discuss Joseph's medical history, which is unremarkable. His only travel has been a hiking trip to the Great Smoky Mountains in East Tennessee approximately 3 months ago. Joseph states he remembers removing a tick from his back after returning home. Upon assessment, Joseph is fatigued, diaphoretic, tachycardic, febrile, and has a small red rash spreading over his trunk. Blood work as well as blood cultures are performed, and all tests are negative. Could Joseph have Lyme disease?

The actions of the nurse in retrieving a thorough history and performing a thorough physical examination may reveal important information in Joseph's case. The hiking trip exposed Joseph to the possibility of a tick bite; however, Tennessee is not listed in the Lyme endemic area. Would you consider this Lyme disease?

Southern tick-associated rash illness

Although Tennessee is not in the classic Lyme disease region where *Borrelia burgdorferi* thrives, another spirochete is now being mentioned in the literature [14–16]. STARI presents with symptomology similar to that of Lyme disease [14–16]. A typical erythema migrans rash can develop as well as mild flulike symptoms. Blood tests and cerebral fluid tests have been negative for all but one patient. The tick believed to be the carrier of this spirochete is *Amblyomma americanum* or the Lone Star tick, which is endogenous to the southeastern region of the United States. *Borrelia lonestari* is thought to be the spirochete involved [17].

The critical care nurse must inquire about the travel, work, and play habits of the patient as well as inspecting the patient's skin thoroughly. Both the history and physical examination will assist in ruling out the existence of both Lyme disease and

STARI. The etiology of STARI is presently unknown, and diagnosis follows much the same course as that for Lyme disease [15]. STARI has been shown to respond quickly to antibiotic therapy with no residual effects. The National Institute of Allergy and Infectious Diseases at the National Institutes of Health, along with the Centers for Disease Control, continues to investigate this occurrence and encourages health care practitioners to submit samples from patients who have the symptoms of STARI to the Centers for Disease Control for continued study. The symptoms are real, and the patient is suffering and seeking help. Continued investigative efforts eventually will demonstrate the etiology and pathophysiology so that treatment can occur and the patient can find relief.

Web sites of interest not cited in the article

American Lyme Disease Foundation, Inc. http://www.aldf.com/.

The Lyme Disease Foundation. http://www.lyme.org.

National institutes of Arthritis and Musculoskeletal and Skin Diseases. National Institutes of Health. http://www.niams.nih.gov.

References

[1] Centers for Disease Control and Prevention. Reported Lyme disease cases by state, 1993–2005. Available at: http://www.cdc.gov/ncidod/dvbid/lyme/ld_rptdLymeCasesbyState.htm. Accessed December 15, 2006.

[2] Sigal LH. Epidemiology and clinical manifestations of Lyme disease. Up To Date. Available at: http://www.uptodateonline.com/application/topic/print.asp?file=othr_inf/6836&type=A&s. Accessed July 30, 2004.

[3] Centers for Disease Control and Prevention. Lyme disease. Available at: http://www.cdc.gov/ncidod/dvbid/lyme/index.htm. Accessed December 15, 2006.

[4] Sigal LH. Bacteriology and epidemiology of Lyme disease. Up To Date. Available at: http://www.uptodateonline.com/utd/content/topic.do?topicKey=tickflea/7074&view=print. Accessed April 25, 2006.

[5] Centers for Disease Control and Prevention. Reported clinical findings among Lyme disease patients. Available at: http://www.cdc.gov/ncidod/dvbid/lyme/ld_bysymptoms.htm. Accessed September 22, 2006.

[6] Sigal LH. Immunopathogenesis of Lyme disease. Up To Date. Available at: http://www.uptodateonline.com/utd/content/topic.do?topicKey=tickflea/9378&view=print. Accessed April 25, 2006.

[7] National Institute of Allergy and Infectious Disease. National Institutes of Health. NIAID Research. Co-infection. Available at: http://www.niaid.nih.gov/research/topics/lyme/research/co-infection/. Accessed September 22, 2006.

[8] Wormser GP, Nadelman RJ, Dattwyler RJ, et al. Practice guidelines for the treatment of Lyme disease. Clin Infect Dis 2000;31(Suppl 1):S1–14.

[9] White DJ, Talarico J, Chang H-G, et al. Human babesiosis in New York State: review of 139 hospitalized cases and analysis of prognostic factors. Arch Intern Med 1998;158:2149–54.

[10] Bakken JS, Krueth J, Wilson-Nordskog C, et al. Clinical and laboratory characteristics of human granulocytic ehrlichiosis. JAMA 1996;275:199–205.

[11] Bransfield PS, Sherr V, Smith H, et al. Evaluation of antibiotic treatment in patients with persistent symptoms of Lyme disease: an ILADS position paper. Bethesda (MD): The International Lyme and Associated Diseases Society; 2003.

[12] Centers for Disease Control and Prevention. Lyme disease diagnosis. Available at: http://www.cdc.gov/ncidod/dvbid/lyme/ld_humandisease_diagnosis.htm. Accessed April 25, 2006.

[13] Gilbert DN, Moellering RC, Eliopoulos GM, et al. The Sanford guide to antimicrobial therapy. 36th edition. Hyde Park (VT): Merck; 2006.

[14] Centers for Disease Control and Prevention. Lone Star tick a concern, but not for Lyme disease. Available at: http://www.cdc.gov/ncidod/dvbid/stari/stari_LoneStarConcern.html. Accessed September 22, 2006.

[15] Sexton DJ. Southern tick-associated rash illness (STARI). 2006. Up To Date. Available at: http://www.uptodateonline.com/utd/content/topic.do?topicKey=tickflea/11896&view=print. Accessed April 25, 2006.

[16] Centers for Disease Control and Prevention. Southern tick-associated rash illness. Available at: http://www.cdc.gov/ncidod/dvbid/stari/index.htm. Accessed December 15, 2006.

[17] James AM, Liveris D, Wormser GP, et al. Borrelia lonestari infection after a bite by an Amblyomma americanum tick. J Infect Dis 2001;183:1810–4.

ELSEVIER
SAUNDERS

Crit Care Nurs Clin N Am 19 (2007) 43–51

CRITICAL CARE
NURSING CLINICS
OF NORTH AMERICA

Antimicrobials: Classifications and Uses in Critical Care

Francisca Cisneros-Farrar, EdD, RN[a,b,*],
Lynn C. Parsons, DSN, RN, CNA-BC[c]

[a]School of Nursing, Austin Peay State University, McCord Building, Room 128, PO Box 4658,
Clarksville, TN 37044, USA
[b]Neurology Intensive Care Unit, St. Thomas Hospital, 4220 Harding Road, Nashville, TN 37205, USA
[c]School of Nursing, Middle Tennessee State University, Box 81, Murfreesboro, TN 37132, USA

Patients admitted to critical care are in a crisis situation. It is common to receive a patient to the unit who has been life-flighted with multisystem failure. It is also common to receive a patient after trauma or emergency surgery. Every second counts as emergency measures are implemented to save the person's life and preserve residual function of the person. Many health care professionals await the arrival of the patient. Emergency measures include intubation with ventilator support for respiratory failure, central line placement, arterial line placement, Foley catheter placement, and immediate diagnostic tests. With all these emergency interventions, the person's normal host defenses are breached or at least compromised, which makes the person vulnerable to infection.

Clinically, the person may present with an active infection, and at the least, the patient is at high risk to develop an infection as a comorbidity or hospital-acquired infection. A vigilant nurse monitors the patient's temperature, vital signs, and white blood cell count to intervene early in the infection cycle. The critical care patient presenting with any infectious process is in a life-threatening situation. The knowledgeable nurse can use interventions that can save the patient's life. At the first sign of infection, cultures

must be done, including urinalysis, blood cultures, and cultures from the site of suspected infection, and a chest radiograph must be taken immediately. The physician needs to be notified without delay for the implementation of these early standards of care for infection. The patient is started on a broad-spectrum antibiotic, such as vancomycin, for empiric therapy, because culture results typically take up to 72 hours. When the microorganism is confirmed, the patient can be changed to the correct antimicrobial that matches the pathogen. Frequently, a referral is made to an infection control physician for consultation on the most effective antimicrobial to be used in critical care patients. Furthermore, the infection control nurse should be consulted and be an active member of the team developing the patient's plan of care.

Purpose

This article reviews antibacterial, antifungal, and antiviral drugs commonly used in the critical care unit. Classifications are identified, with examples given for commonly used drugs in the critical care setting. Common adverse effects, serious adverse effects, and toxicity signals are identified in an effort to educate the nurse in preventing these effects and maximizing the benefits of antimicrobial drugs. In some cases, multiple antimicrobials may be needed to combat infection. These scenarios commonly become more complex with the possibility of high risks

* Corresponding author. Austin Peay State University, McCord Building, Room 128, PO Box 4658, Clarksville, TN 37044.

E-mail address: farrarf@apsu.edu (F. Cisneros-Farrar).

for toxicity of drugs because of renal, cardiac, and hepatic impairment of the patient; drug interactions attributable to multiple intravenous medications being used to treat the patient; and risks for suprainfections. Suprainfections signal the emergence of patient drug resistance [1]. Antimicrobial agents are usually given intravenously in the critical care setting because of the acuity and complexity of the infection. Occasionally, an antimicrobial may be given by means of an oral gastric tube, nasogastric tube, or Dobbhoff tube.

β-Lactam antibacterials

The β-lactam antibiotics are named after their chemical structure, which includes a β-lactam ring that is essential for antibacterial activity [2]. These antibiotics inhibit synthesis of bacterial cell walls by binding to proteins in bacterial cell membranes, causing intracellular contents to leak from the cell. This destruction of microorganisms is most effective when bacterial cells are dividing [3]. β-lactam antibiotics have four major subclasses: penicillins, cephalosporins, carbapems, and monobactams [3].

Penicillins

Penicillins can be classified into four major subgroups based on their structure and the spectrum of bacteria they destroy: natural penicillins, penicillinase-resistant penicillins, aminopenicillins, and extended-spectrum penicillins [4]. Penicillin–β-lactamase inhibitors are a combination drug of penicillin and a β-lactamase inhibitor that protects the penicillin from destruction by enzymes [3]. Penicillin is a natural agent obtained from the mold genus *Penicillium*. This classification includes natural extracts from the *Penicillium* mold, such as the fungus or mold often seen on bread or fruit [5].

Penicillin was introduced during World War II and saved many soldiers' lives. Penicillin G and penicillin V were labeled miracle drugs and were widely used. The overuse of penicillin to treat staphylococcal infections caused mutant strains of *Staphylococcus* to develop that were resistant to penicillin G and penicillin V. This led to the development of new broad-spectrum antibiotics similar to penicillin to combat infections [6]. Penicillins are most commonly used for gram-positive bacteria, including *Streptococcus*, *Enterococcus*, and *Staphylococcus* [2]. Penicillins are often used in urinary tract infections, wound infections,

respiratory infections, and gastrointestinal infections [5]. In the critical care setting, where patients may have multiple organism or nosocomial infections, the extended-spectrum drugs and penicillin–β-lactamase inhibitor combinations are most likely to be used [7].

Penicillin G is an example of a natural penicillin. It remains the drug of choice for the treatment of streptococcal pharyngitis [3]. Penicillin G should not be injected intravenously or mixed with other intravenous solutions because of the drug's association with cardiorespiratory arrest and death [8]. Penicillin G is most commonly used in the critical care setting to treat streptococcal group A bacterial upper respiratory infections [7]. Penicillin G is frequently used for a variety of anaerobes that have an affinity for the human mouth. Left untreated, these anaerobes can trigger nosocomial aspiration pneumonia [7]. It is also used to treat active streptococcal endocarditis. The drug is to be administered intramuscularly in the upper outer quadrant of the buttock. Before administration, a culture should be done to identify *Streptococcus* as the causative agent of the infection [4]. The nurse should monitor the patient's renal function, mental status, vital signs, and complete blood cell count (CBC) [8]. Penicillin G is contraindicated in patients with a past history of hypersensitivity to any of the penicillins. Precautions should be taken if the patient has a history of allergies or asthma. Common adverse reactions are rash, urticaria, and fever. Serious and potentially life-threatening adverse reactions are edema of the larynx and anaphylaxis [8].

Penicillinase-resistant penicillins are a group of antibiotics that are effective in the treatment of infections caused by staphylococci resistant to penicillin G. These antibiotics are not used for treatment of methicillin-resistant *Staphylococcus aureus* (MRSA) infections [3]. Nafcillin (Unipen) is an example of a drug used in the critical care setting [7]. It is most commonly used for severe endocarditis. The usual dose should be reduced by 50% for patients with severe renal and hepatic impairment [9]. Nafcillin may also be given intraperitoneally in the treatment of dialysis-associated peritonitis. The nurse should monitor the patient's CBC with assessment of the differential, electrolytes, liver function, and renal function. A serious adverse effect is hypokalemia and interstitial nephritis. A major drug interaction occurs with cyclosporine. Moderate drug interactions occur with nifedipine and warfarin [9].

Ampicillin (Principen) is an example of an aminopenicillin. Ampicillin is a broad-spectrum semisynthetic penicillin [3]. Ampicillin is used to treat bacterial infections caused by susceptible streptococci, *Streptococcus pneumoniae*, non–penicillase-producing staphylococci, meningococci, *Listeria, Klebsiella, Escherichia coli, Haemophilus influenzae, Salmonella*, and *Shigella* [10]. It is used in the critical setting to treat respiratory tract infections, meningitis, infection of the genitourinary tract, and infection of the digestive system [7]. The nurse should monitor the patient's CBC and renal function. In streptococcal infections, a culture should be done at the completion of the ampicillin therapy [10]. Common adverse effects are rash, urticaria, diarrhea, nausea, and vomiting. A serious adverse effect is a hypersensitivity reaction. Drug interactions can occur with ethinyl, estradiol, etonogestrel, khat, mestranol, norelgestromin, norethindrone, and norgestrel [10].

Extended-spectrum penicillins are broad-spectrum antibiotics that are effective against gram-negative organisms, such as *Pseudomonas, Proteus*, and *E coli* [4]. In the critical care setting, the extended-spectrum drugs and penicillin–β-lactamase inhibitor combinations are most likely to be used [3]. This combination extends the antimicrobial spectrum of the penicillins. These drugs are available in fixed-dose combinations with penicillin. Three common combination formulations available parenterally are ampicillin/sulbactam (Unasyn), ticarcillin/clavulanate (Timentin), and piperacillin/tazobactam (Zosyn) [7].

These agents can be effective in the treatment of mixed infections. In settings in which there is overwhelming infection by gram-negative bacilli, extended-spectrum penicillins should not be used as a single-agent therapy. An aminoglycoside should be administered concomitantly to provide broader gram-negative coverage [7]. A common combination used in the critical care unit is piperacillin/tazobactam (Zosyn) [4]. An aminoglycoside is usually given concomitantly to provide broader gram-negative coverage [7]. Piperacillin/tazobactam (Zosyn) is used to treat bacterial infections caused by gram-positive and gram-negative aerobic and anaerobic microorganisms [4]. It is commonly used to treat community-acquired pneumonia, nosocomial pneumonia, appendicitis, infection of skin and subcutaneous tissue, peritonitis, and pelvic disease [4]. Doses should be adjusted for patients with renal disease [2]. The nurse should monitor the patient's CBC by assessment of the differential, renal function, serum electrolytes, and liver function [4]. High doses of piperacillin/tazobactam (Zosyn) are associated with seizure activity, especially in patients with renal impairment [4]. There is also a risk for bleeding manifestations in patients with renal impairment. Additional precautions should be taken in patients requiring sodium restriction [11]. Common adverse effects are pruritus, rash, diarrhea, nausea, vomiting, and headache. A serious adverse reaction is an allergic reaction leading to anaphylaxis. Piperacillin/tozobactam (Zosyn) has a drug interaction with methotrexate and vecuronium [11].

Cephalosporins

Cephalosporins are semisynthetic antibiotic derivatives of cephalosporin C, which is a substance produced by a fungus and altered synthetically to produce an antibiotic [2]. In 1948, a fungus called *Cephalosporium acremonium* was discovered in seawater at a sewer outlet. The fungus was found to be active against gram-positive and gram-negative microorganisms and resistant to β-lactamase [6]. Cephalosporin molecules were chemically altered, and semisynthetic cephalosporins were produced to increase broader spectrum antibiotics [6]. Cephalosporins are broad-spectrum antibiotics effective against gram-positive and gram-negative bacteria. These antibiotics are used in the treatment of bloodstream, brain, spinal cord, urinary tract, respiratory, skin and soft tissue, bone, and joint infections [3]. Cephalosporins are classified as first, second, third, and fourth generations [12].

First-generation drugs are often used for surgical prophylaxis [3]. Cefazolin (Ancef) is frequently used as a parenteral agent in the critical care setting. Second-generation drugs are frequently used for treatment of intra-abdominal infections [3]. Cefuroxime axetil (Ceftin) is used as a parenteral agent in the critical care setting. Third-generation drugs are recommended for serious infections, such as those caused by *E coli* and *Proteus, Klebsiella*, and *Serratia* species [5]. Ceftriaxone (Rocephin) is frequently used as a parenteral agent in the critical care setting. Fourth-generation drugs are used to treat serious gram-negative infections [3]. Fourth-generation drugs have increased activity against gram-positive cocci and gram-negative bacilli [5]. Cefepime (Maxipime) is frequently used as a parenteral agent in the critical care setting. This drug is the most commonly used cephalosporin in the critical care setting. Cefepime (Maxipime) is a semisynthetic antibiotic that is used to treat a wide range of gram-positive and gram-negative bacteria [2]. It is commonly used for empiric therapy for febrile neutropenia. It is also used to treat complicated infections in the abdomen, pneumonia, genitourinary infections, and infections of the skin or subcutaneous tissue [3]. Dose adjustment should be considered for patients with renal impairment [13]. The nurse should monitor the patient's CBC, hepatic and liver function, antibiotic-associated diarrhea, signs of serum sickness–like reactions, and prothrombin time. Common adverse reactions are rash, colitis, diarrhea, dyspepsia, and headache. Serious neurologic adverse reactions are myoclonus and seizure [13]. Acute renal impairment can occur without dose adjustment.

Carbapenems

Carbapenems are broad-spectrum antibiotics and consist of three current drugs: imipenem-cilastatin (Primaxin), meropenem (Merrem), and ertapenem (Invanz) [3]. Carbapenems are usually used as a last resort. They are usually reserved for complicated body cavity and connective tissue infections in critically ill patients. A serious adverse effect is drug-induced seizure activity [3]. When receiving this medication, the patient should be placed on seizure precautions.

Imipenem-cilastatin (Primaxin) is a common parenteral drug used in the critical care setting [3]. This antibiotic is used to treat severe life-threatening bacterial infections caused by gram-negative multiple organism infections, gram-positive organisms, and anaerobic organisms [2]. It is used to treat lower respiratory tract infections, infections of the abdomen, infections of the skin or subcutaneous tissue, and complicated urinary tract infections [12]. Dose adjustment needs to be made for patients with renal impairment and for adult patients who weigh less than 70 kg [6]. The nurse should monitor the patient's CBC. Common adverse effects are thrombophlebitis, diarrhea, nausea, and vomiting [3]. Serious adverse effects are seizure, renal impairment, and anaphylaxis. Drug interactions occur with ganciclovir, theophylline, and cyclosporine [14].

Meropenem (Merrem IV) is a β-lactam carbapenem antibiotic that is commonly used in the critical setting to treat systemic infections caused by gram-positive and gram-negative bacteria [7].

Meropenem has a strong affinity toward *E coli*, *Pseudomonas*, and *S aureus* [12]. Meropenem is used clinically to treat bacterial meningitis, complicated infections of the abdomen, and complicated infections of the skin or subcutaneous tissue [2]. The nurse should monitor the patient's CBC, renal function, and hepatic function. Common adverse effects are diarrhea, nausea, and headache. Serious adverse effects include erythema, Stevens-Johnson syndrome, toxic epidermal necrosis, agranulocytosis, leukopenia, neutropenia, seizure, and angioedema. A moderate drug interaction occurs with valproic acid [7].

Ertapenem sodium (Invanz) is another common parental β-lactam carbapenem used in the critical care setting [7]. This antibiotic is used in the treatment of gram-positive and gram-negative aerobes and anaerobes [12]. Clinically, it is used to treat community-acquired pneumonia, diabetic foot infections without osteomyelitis, complicated infections of the skin or subcutaneous tissue, complicated infections of the abdomen, and complicated urinary tract infections [15]. The nurse should monitor the patient's CBC and hepatic function [3]. Common adverse effects are diarrhea, nausea, vomiting, vaginitis, and headache. Serious adverse effects are disturbance of consciousness and seizure [8]. A moderate drug interaction occurs with probenecid [15].

Monobactams

Monobactams are bactericidal agents that are used in the treatment of gram-negative bacteria [12]. They have similar activity as β-lactam antibiotics and cephalosporins [2]. Monobactams have a salient therapeutic advantage because they preserve normal gram-positive and anaerobic flora [2]. Aztreonam (Azactam) is a monobactam antibiotic that is commonly used in the critical care setting. It is a systemic bactericidal used to treat multiple gram-negative bacteria and severe gram-negative septicemia [7]. It is clinically used to treat lower respiratory infections; diseases of the abdomen; respiratory infections, including *Klebsiella pneumoniae* and *H influenzae*; and urinary tract infections [16]. Dose adjustments need to be made for geriatric patients based on renal function and for all patients with renal impairment [7]. The nurse should monitor the patient's CBC [5]. Common adverse effects are rash, diarrhea, nausea, vomiting, and drug-induced eosinophilia [16]. Serious adverse effects are thrombophlebitis, neutropenia, pancytopenia, hepatotoxicity, and anaphylaxis.

On rare occasions, pseudomembranous enterocolitis can occur [16].

Aminoglycosides

The aminoglycosides are a group of natural and semisynthetic antibiotics. Streptomycin sulfate, derived from the bacterium *Streptomyces griseus* in 1944, was the first aminoglycoside available for clinical use and was used to treat tuberculosis [17]. Aminoglycosides are used to treat infections caused by gram-negative microorganisms, such as *Pseudomonas*, *Proteus*, *Klebsiella*, *Enterobacter*, and *Serratia* species and *E coli* [18]. Parental aminoglycosides are used to treat serious systemic infections caused by susceptible aerobic gram-negative organisms [19]. Toxicity limits are used to treat serious gram-negative infections and specific conditions involving gram-positive cocci [5]. Critical care patients are at high risk for developing ototoxicity and nephrotoxicity, particularly at these high doses. Dosage reductions should be made based on renal function [19]. Peak and trough drug levels should be measured to prevent toxicity [5]. Suprainfection of candidiasis and pseudomembranous colitis can occur [5]. Aminoglycosides are usually given with other antibiotics to provide broad-spectrum activity. The three most commonly used aminoglycosides for the treatment of systemic infections are amikacin, gentamicin, and tobramycin [2].

Fluoroquinolones

These antibiotics are used for the treatment of gram-negative and gram-positive organisms. Fluoroquinolones are potent broad-spectrum antibiotics that destroy bacteria by altering DNA [2]. Ciprofloxacin (Cipro) and levofloxacin (Levaquin) are two common parental fluoroquinolones used in the critical care setting [7]. Ciprofloxacin (Cipro) is an antibiotic used to treat infection caused by *E coli*, *K pneumoniae*, *Enterobacter cloacae*, *Proteus mirabilis*, *H influenzae*, *Moraxella catarrhalis*, *Staphylococcus pneumoniae*, *S aureus*, *Streptococcus pyogenes*, *Campylobacter jejuni*, *Shigella* species, and *Salmonella typhi* [2]. It is used as empiric therapy in the treatment of febrile neutropenia [20]. It is also used to treat bone infections, infections of the skin or subcutaneous tissue, infectious diarrheal diseases, infections of abdomen, lower respiratory infections, nosocomial pneumonia, sinusitis, and urinary tract infections. It has most recently been brought to the attention of the American public because of its use as prophylaxis for or treatment of postexposure inhalation anthrax [20]. Dose adjustment needs to be made for patients with renal impairment [2]. The nurse should monitor the patient's CBC and renal function [8]. Common adverse effects are rash, diarrhea, nausea, dizziness, headache, and restlessness [20]. Serious adverse effects are hypersensitivity reaction, tendonitis with rare rupture of the tendon, peripheral neuropathy, raised intracranial pressure, seizure, and drug-induced psychosis [20]. There are multiple drug interactions with ciprofloxacin (Cipro) [20].

Levofloxacin (Levaquin) is a parental drug frequently given in the critical care setting. It is a systemic fluoroquinolone antibiotic [7]. It is used in the critical care setting to treat bronchitis, community-acquired pneumonia, nosocomial pneumonia, urinary tract infections, infections of skin or subcutaneous tissue, and bacterial sinusitis [21]. It is also used as prophylaxis after exposure of inhalant anthrax [21]. As with most antibiotics, the dose should be adjusted in patients with renal impairment [5]. The nurse should monitor the patient's CBC, paying special attention to the white blood cell count. Common adverse effects are diarrhea, nausea, headache, and blurred vision [21]. Serious adverse effects are torsades de pointes, hyperglycemia or hypoglycemia in diabetic patients, hypersensitivity reaction, tendon rupture, and polyneuropathy [21]. There are multiple drug interactions with levofloxacin (Levaquin), including such common medications as glyburide, metformin, and insulins. A thorough assessment of the medications any patient is taking is always indicated, but because of the many interactions with Levaquin, this is particularly imperative [21].

Macrolides and ketolides

Macrolides are a large group of antibiotics that were introduced in the early 1950s with erythromycin [5]. Macrolides are broad-spectrum antibiotics. Erythromycin was the first drug introduced and was derived from the fungus-like bacteria *Streptomyces erythreus* [17]. Macrolides are effective against gram-positive cocci, including group A streptococci, pneumococci, and staphylococci [22].

Erythromycin is a macrolide antibiotic used to treat respiratory tract infection caused by

Mycoplasma pneumoniae, intestinal infections caused by Entamoeba histolytica, chlamydial infection, bacterial lower respiratory infection caused by S pyogenes or S pneumonia, Legionnaire's disease, and listeriosis [23]. It is also used as a penicillin substitute in patients who are allergic to penicillin [22]. Doses need to be adjusted for patients with hepatic impairment [24]. The nurse should monitor the patient's white blood cell count. Common adverse effects are diarrhea, loss of appetite, nausea, stomach cramps, vomiting, and decreased liver function [23]. Serious adverse reactions are cardiac dysrhythmia, torsades de pointes, pyloric stenosis, hearing loss, ototoxicity, and anaphylaxis [23]. There are multiple drug interactions with erythromycin [23].

Other antibiotic treatments

Clindamycin (Cleocin HCl) is a lincosamide antibiotic used to treat bacterial infections caused by the anaerobic organisms staphylococci, streptococci, and pneumococci [25]. It is used to treat infections of the skin or subcutaneous tissue, infections of abdomen, and lower respiratory infections [22]. Clindamycin can cause diarrhea, colitis, and pseudomembranes colitis [24]. It is used judiciously in the critical care setting because of its promulgation of hepatic impairment and antibiotic-associated diarrhea [22]. Use of this drug is of particular concern when a patient presents with severe colitis, because this medication may contribute to death in patients who present with diarrhea before antibiotic therapy [25]. Dose adjustment needs to be made for patients with hepatic impairment who exhibit severe liver disease [2]. The nurse should monitor the patient's CBC, liver function, kidney function, and diarrhea [24]. Common adverse effects are rash, diarrhea, and nausea. Serious adverse effects are increased liver function on testing, jaundice, and pseudomembranous enterocolitis [25]. Drug interactions occur with erythromycin, atracurium, cyclosporine, metocurine, and tubocurarine [25].

Linezolid (Zyvox) is a new antibiotic in the oxalodinone class that is used to treat aerobic gram-positive bacteria [22]. This systemic antibiotic is used to treat community-acquired pneumonia and diseases caused by gram-positive bacteria, including MRSA strains, nosocomial pneumonia, vancomycin-resistant Enterococcus faecium (VREF) infection, and infection of skin or subcutaneous tissue [26]. Linezolid is a weak monoamine

oxidase inhibitor; thus, foods high in tyramine content should be avoided [22]. Foods like aged or dried meats and poultry, cheeses, nuts, and all alcoholic or fermented beverages contain high amounts of tyramine. The patient's CBC warrants weekly monitoring, as do signs and symptoms of lactic acidosis and visual impairment [26]. Common adverse effects are diarrhea, nausea, and headache [24]. Serious side effects are myelosuppression, peripheral neuropathy, and optic neuropathy [26].

Vancomycin hydrochloride (Vancomycin) is a tricyclic glycopeptide antibiotic that is used to treat several aerobic and anaerobic gram-positive bacteria [27]. It is used clinically to treat bacterial infections caused by strains of S aureus [2]. Vancomycin hydrochloride is used frequently parentally in the critical care setting to treat infections caused by MRSA and methicillin-resistant staphylococcal species non-aureus (SSNA) [22]. It is also used to treat endocarditis, meningitis, and antibiotic-associated pseudomembranous colitis (Clostridium difficile) [12,27]. Vancomycin hydrochloride is used in the treatment of infections with susceptible organisms in patients allergic to penicillins [12]. Vancomycin hydrochloride reaches therapeutic plasma levels within 1 hour after infusion. If the drug is given too rapidly, an adverse reaction caused by a histamine-associated reaction known as "redneck syndrome" can occur. This syndrome is manifested by flushing, skin rash over the upper trunk and face, hypotension, tingling, pruritus, and hypotension [7]. For patients with renal impairment and anuria, the dose should be adjusted. The nurse should monitor the patient's CBC with assessment of the differential, renal function, signs and symptoms of ototoxicity, and therapeutic trough and peak levels to prevent toxicity [12]. Common adverse effects are drug-induced erythroderma, nausea, and vomiting [27]. Serious adverse effects are neutropenia, ototoxicity, nephrotoxicity, and anaphylaxis [27]. Gentamicin, amikacin, succinylcholine, and warfarin are prone to cause drug interactions [27].

Dalfopristin/quinupristin (Synercid) is a systemic antibiotic that is used to treat bacteremia caused by VREF infection and complicated skin or subcutaneous tissue infections caused by Staphylococcus and Streptococcus species bacteria [28]. This drug had an accelerated approval, and ongoing research is being conducted to validate traditional clinical end points to dalfopristin/quinupristin's clinical benefit [28]. Dose adjustment needs to be made for persons with liver disease [7]. The nurse should monitor the patient's CBC and bilirubin levels [28]. Common adverse effects are thrombophlebitis, rash, diarrhea, nausea, vomiting, hyperbilirubinemia, arthralgia, myalgia, and headache [28]. There are multiple drug interactions [28].

Antifungal agents

Fungi are large and diverse microorganisms that include all yeasts and molds. The infection caused by a fungus is called mycosis. Fungal infections can be systemic and life threatening. In persons with a compromised immune system, such as critical care patients, the risk for developing fungal infections is high. The use of antibiotics and immunosuppressants, such as corticosteroids, may cause colonization of *Candida albicans*, which can lead to a systemic infection [29]. Amphotericin B is the agent of choice for the treatment of severe systemic mycoses in the critical care setting [29]. Metronidazole (Flagyl) and fluconazole (Diflucan) are also used to treat fungal infections in the critical care setting [7].

Amphotericin B (Amphocin) is a polyene antifungal agent used to treat systemic progressive and potentially life-threatening fungal infections [30]. The drug should not be used for the treatment of noninvasive forms of fungal disease [31]. In the critical setting, amphotericin B is used to treat potentially life-threatening systemic mycosis fungal infections, fungal infections of the lung, fungal infections of the central nervous system, candidiasis of the skin, and urinary tract mycosis [7,31]. It is usually given over a long-term period from 4 to 12 weeks. Fever, chills, hypotension, and tachypnea are the most common symptoms of an infusion reaction [32]. Pretreatment with acetaminophen, hydrocortisone, or meperidine can ameliorate the incidence and severity of these symptoms [7]. For patients with renal impairment, the dose must be monitored and adjusted. The nurse should monitor the patient for negative cultures for specific fungi, CBC, hepatic function, renal function, and serum electrolytes [31]. Common adverse effects over the long course of treatment include weight loss, diarrhea, dyspepsia, loss of appetite, nausea, vomiting, chills, fever, headache, and malaise [31]. Serious adverse effects are hypotension, thrombophlebitis, hypokalemia, anemia, thrombocytopenia, anaphylaxis, seizure, blurred vision, double vision, nephrotoxicity, and tachypnea [31]. A drug interaction occurs with cyclosporine [31]. Although lipid formulations of amphotericin B, such as Abelcet and Amphotec, have been developed to decrease renal toxicity, nephrotoxicity remains the most serious long-term adverse effect [7]. The lipid formulations are more expensive but can deliver a higher dose and increased therapeutic effects [7].

Itraconazole (Sporanox) is a broad-spectrum azole antifungal agent that is effective for blastomycosis, histoplasmosis, paracoccidioidomycosis, and sporotrichosis [7]. It is an alternative to amphotericin B for aspergillosis, candidiasis, and coccidioidomycosis [30]. Itraconazole has two potentially serious side effects: cardiac suppression and liver injury [30]. Because critical care patients are particularly vulnerable to these effects, the benefits of using this medication should have empiric evidence that its use outweighs the risks [30].

Fluconazole (Diflucan) is a triazole antifungal agent that is used to treat candidiasis with bone marrow transplantation, candidiasis of the esophagus, candiduria, cryptococcal meningitis, disseminated candidiasis, and oral candidiasis [32]. For patients with renal impairment, the dose should be adjusted accordingly [30]. In addition to renal function, the nurse should monitor the patient's electrocardiogram (ECG), hepatic function, and exfoliative skin disorders [32]. Common adverse effects are pruritus, rash, nausea, vomiting, increased liver enzymes, and headache. A serious adverse effect is anaphylaxis [32]. There are multiple drug interactions [32].

Antiviral drugs

The two major categories of antiviral drugs are (1) *antiviral agents*, which is a general term for agents used to treat infections caused by viruses other than HIV, and (2) *antiretroviral agents*, which is a general term for agents used to treat infections caused by HIV [29]. A common antiviral drug used in the critical setting is acyclovir (Zovirax) [7].

Acyclovir (Zovirax) is an antiviral agent that is a viral DNA polymerase inhibitor and a guanosine nucleoside analogue [33]. Acyclovir is used to treat herpes simplex, herpes zoster, varicella, and herpes simplex encephalitis [34]. The dose warrants adjustment based on the weight of the patient (particularly those who are obese) and for patients with renal impairment [33]. The nurse should monitor the patient's renal function [29]. A common adverse effect of the topical form of Zovirax is a burning sensation of the skin to which the medication is applied. Parenteral and enteral forms of the medication have adverse effects, such as diarrhea, nausea, vomiting, agitation, confusion, dizziness, hallucination, elevated serum blood urea nitrogen, elevated serum creatinine, and malaise [33]. Serious adverse effects are thrombocytopenic purpura, confusion, encephalopathic changes, lethargy, tremor, agitation, hemolytic uremic syndrome, and renal impairment [33]. Drug interactions occur with varicella virus vaccine, fosphenytoin, phenytoin, and valproic acid [33].

Valacyclovir (Valtrex) is a prodrug form of acyclovir. This antiviral drug is used for treatment of infection with herpes simplex viruses and varicella zoster virus [34]. Drug benefits depend on the conversion of valacyclovir to acyclovir, which is its active form [34]. Acyclovir or valacyclovir is used prophylactically for patients who are undergoing bone marrow or solid organ transplantation [7].

Summary

Patients in the critical care setting are at high risk for infection because their normal host defenses are compromised. Critical care patients frequently have complicated, multisystem, mixed infections that can be life threatening. Optimal patient outcomes are the result of (1) early identification of signs and symptoms of infection; (2) nursing knowledge about common antimicrobials and their side effects and adverse reactions; (3) obtaining cultures before starting empiric therapy with antimicrobials; (4) consulting as needed with the infection control team; (5) practicing basic measures of infection control, such as hand washing; and (6) using special isolation precautions when the patient's condition warrants special care. The nurse also needs to be vigilant to the signs of toxicity from antimicrobial therapy. These interventions can save the critical care patient's life, prevent others from becoming infected, and save the hospital precious fiscal resources.

References

[1] Lehne RA. Basic principles of antimicrobial therapy. In: Pharmacology for nursing care. St. Louis (MO): Sanders Elsevier; 2007. p. 948–61.

[2] Lilley LL, Scott H, Synder J. Antibiotics. In: Pharmacology and the nursing process. 4th edition. St. Louis (MO): Mosby; 2005. p. 619–53.

[3] Abrams AC, Pennington SS, Lammon CB. Beta-lactam antibacterials: penicillins, cephalosporins, and other drugs. In: Clinical drug therapy rationales for nursing practice. 8th edition. Philadelphia: Lippincott Williams and Wilkins; 2007. p. 485–503.

[4] Lehne RA. Drugs that weaken the bacterial cell wall I: penicillins. In: Pharmacology for nursing care. St. Louis (MO): Sanders Elsevier; 2007. p. 962–71.

[5] Hogan MA. Anti-infective medications. In: Prentice Hall nursing pharmacology reviews and rationale. Upper Saddle River (NJ): Pearson Prentice Hall; 2005. p. 25–98.

[6] Kee JL, Hayes ER, McCaistion LE. Antibacterials: penicillins and cephalosporins. In: Pharmacology: a nursing process approach. 5th edition. St. Louis (MO): Sanders Elsevier; 2006. p. 423–38.

[7] Daly JS, Glew RH. Use of antimicrobials in the treatment of infection in the critically ill patient. In: Irwin RS, Rippe JM, editors. Irwin and Rippe's intensive care medicine. 5th edition. Philadelphia: Lippincott Williams and Wilkins; 2003. p. 1–36. Ovid electronic textbook. Available at: http://gateway.ut.ovid.com/gwl/ovidweb.cg. Accessed January 28, 2006.

[8] Thompson Micromedex from Micromedex Health Care Series. Drug point summary penicillin benzathine. Available at: http://www.thomsonhc.com/hcs/librarian/ND-PR/Main. Accessed July 28, 2006.

[9] Thompson Micromedex from Micromedex Health Care Series. Drug point summary nafcillin sodium. Available at: http://www.thomsonhc.com/hcs/librarian/ND-PR/Main. Accessed July 28, 2006.

[10] Thompson Micromedex from Micromedex Health Care Series. Drug point summary ampicillin. Available at: http://www.thomsonhc.com/hcs/librarian/ND-PR/Main. Accessed July 28, 2006.

[11] Thompson Micromedex from Micromedex Health Care Series. Drug point summary piperacillin sodium/tazobactam sodium. Available at: http://www.thomsonhc.com/hcs/librarian/ND-PR/Main. Accessed July 28, 2006.

[12] Lehne RA. Drugs that weaken the bacterial cell wall II: cephalosporins, carbapenems, vancomycin, aztreonam, teicoplanin, and fosfomycin. In: Pharmacology for nursing care. St. Louis (MO): Sanders Elsevier; 2007. p. 972–80.

[13] Thompson Micromedex from Micromedex Health Care Series. Drug point summary cefepime hydrochloride. Available at: http://www.thomsonhc.com/hcs/librarian/ND-PR/Main. Accessed July 28, 2006.

[14] Thompson Micromedex from Micromedex Health Care Series. Drug point summary imipenem/cilastatin. Available at: http://www.thomsonhc.com/hcs/librarian/ND-PR/Main. Accessed July 28, 2006.

[15] Thompson Micromedex from Micromedex Health Care Series. Drug point summary ertapenem sodium. Available at: http://www.thomsonhc.com/hcs/librarian/ND-PR/Main. Accessed July 28, 2006.

[16] Thompson Micromedex from Micromedex Health Care Series. Drug point summary aztreonam. Available at: http://www.thomsonhc.com/hcs/librarian/ND-PR/Main. Accessed July 28, 2006.

[17] Kee JL, Hayes ER, McCaistion LE. Antibacterials: macrolides, tetracyclines, aminoglycosides, and fluoroquinolones. In: Pharmacology a nursing process approach. 5th edition. St. Louis (MO): Sanders Elsevier; 2006. p. 439–53.

[18] Lehne RA. Aminoglycosides: bactericidal inhibitors of protein synthesis. In: Pharmacology for nursing care. St. Louis (MO): Sanders Elsevier; 2007. p. 994–1001.

[19] Abrams AC, Pennington SS, Lammon CB. Aminoglycosides and fluoroquinolones. In: Clinical drug therapy rationales for nursing practice. 8th edition. Philadelphia: Lippincott Williams and Wilkins; 2007. p. 504–14.

[20] Thompson Micromedex from Micromedex Health Care Series. Drug point summary ciprofloxacin. Available at: http://www.thomsonhc.com/hcs/librarian/ND-PR/Main. Accessed July 28, 2006.

[21] Thompson Micromedex from Micromedex Health Care Series. Drug point summary levofloxacin. Available at: http://www.thomsonhc.com/hcs/librarian/ND-PR/Main. Accessed July 28, 2006.

[22] Abrams AC, Pennington SS, Lammon CB. Macrolides, ketolides, and miscellaneous antibiotics. In: Clinical drug therapy rationales for nursing practice. 8th edition. Philadelphia (PA): Lippincott Williams and Wilkins; 2007. p. 528–9.

[23] Thompson Micromedex from Micromedex Health Care Series. Drug point summary erythromycin. Available at: http://www.thomsonhc.com/hcs/librarian/ND-PR/Main. Accessed July 28, 2006.

[24] Lehne RA. Bacteriostatic inhibitors of protein synthesis: tetracyclines, macrolides, and others. In: Pharmacology for nursing care. St. Louis (MO): Sanders Elsevier; 2007. p. 981–93.

[25] Thompson Micromedex from Micromedex Health Care Series. Drug point summary clindamycin hydrochloride. Available at: http://www.thomsonhc. com/hcs/librarian/ND-PR/Main. Accessed July 28, 2006.

[26] Thompson Micromedex from Micromedex Health Care Series. Drug point summary linezolid. Available at: http://www.thomsonhc.com/hcs/librarian/ND-PR/Main. Accessed July 28, 2006.

[27] Thompson Micromedex from Micromedex Health Care Series. Drug point summary vancomycin hydrochloride. Available at: http://www.thomsonhc.com/hcs/librarian/ND-PR/Main. Accessed July 28, 2006.

[28] Thompson Micromedex from Micromedex Health Care Series. Drug point summary dalfopristin/quinupristin. Available at:. http://www.thomsonhc.com/hcs/librarian/ND-PR/Main. Accessed July 28, 2006.

[29] Lilley LL, Scott H, Synder J. Antifungal agents. In: Pharmacology and the nursing process. 4th edition. St. Louis (MO): Mosby; 2005. p. 689–99.

[30] Lehne RA. Antifungal agents. In: Pharmacology for nursing care. St. Louis (MO): Sanders Elsevier; 2007. p. 1035–41.

[31] Thompson Micromedex from Micromedex Health Care Series. Drug point summary amphotericin B. Available at: http://www.thomsonhc.com/hcs/librarian/ND-PR/Main. Accessed July 28, 2006.

[32] Thompson Micromedex from Micromedex Health Care Series. Drug point summary fluconazole. Available at: http://www.thomsonhc.com/hcs/librarian/ND-PR/Main. Accessed July 28, 2006.

[33] Thompson Micromedex from Micromedex Health Care Series. Drug point summary acyclovir. Available at: http://www.thomsonhc.com/hcs/librarian/ND-PR/Main. Accessed July 28, 2006.

[34] Lehne RA. Antiviral agents I: drugs for non-HIV viral infections. In: Pharmacology for nursing care. St. Louis (MO): Sanders Elsevier; 2007. p. 1048–61.

ELSEVIER
SAUNDERS

CRITICAL CARE
NURSING CLINICS
OF NORTH AMERICA

Crit Care Nurs Clin N Am 19 (2007) 53–60

Antimicrobial Resistance in Critical Care

Maria A. Smith, DSN, RN, CCRN, COI*,
Leigh Ann McInnis, PhD, APRN, FNP

*School of Nursing, Middle Tennessee State University, 1500 Greenland Drive, PO Box 81,
Murfreesboro, TN 37132, USA*

Approximately 2 million individuals contract bacterial infections in United States hospitals every year. Of these, about 90,000 die as a result [1]. Annually, 500,000 to 1 million cases of sepsis in acute care hospitals result from infectious processes. The mortality rate for these patients is between 15% and 30% [2]. Antimicrobial agents play a critical role in the treatment of many diseases and infections, but antimicrobial resistance now complicates the approach to patients in critical care. Antimicrobial-resistant infections are a frequent cause of mortality and morbidity in hospitalized patients, and septicemia is the tenth leading cause of death in the United States [3,4].

Antimicrobial resistance is of particular concern to nurses in critical care units because they administer larger quantities of antimicrobial agents than their counterparts in other parts of the hospital. Antimicrobial use in critical care units can be 10 times greater than in the rest of the hospital [5]. Microbes and critical care units are not strangers. Critical care units are areas where persons are treated because of severe bacteremia resulting from normal flora or foreign microbe invasion. Thus, patients in critical care areas have a greater opportunity to develop difficulties from antimicrobial administration and antimicrobial resistance than do patients in other areas of the hospital [6].

As in the global environment, many factors in critical care units converge to create the dilemma of antimicrobial resistance. Genetic/biologic, physical/environmental, social/political/economic, and ecologic factors are four overlapping categories

representative of the influences on infectious disease and antimicrobial resistance (Fig. 1) [7]. Antimicrobial agents commonly are used in critical care for prophylaxis and treatment of many infectious diseases. In critical care units, several factors converge to increase the incidence and impact of antimicrobial resistance: the increased number of invasive procedures, common use of indwelling devices, a higher population of immunocompromised patients, and an increased workload that involves the need to initiate life-saving interventions urgently. Antimicrobial resistance is a crucial issue.

Antimicrobial resistance

Overuse or misuse of antimicrobial agents (including agricultural use), an increase in the number of resistant bacteria (evolutionary change), and an aging population are associated with the development of antimicrobial resistance [8]. A few examples of antimicrobial-resistant organisms are (1) methicillin-resistant *Staphylococcus aureus*, (2) vancomycin-intermediate *Staphylococcus aureus*, (3) vancomycin-resistant *Staphylococcus aureus*, and (4) drug-resistant *Streptococcus pneumoniae*; many organisms resistant to drugs such as vancomycin, methicillin, and penicillin are known commonly by their abbreviations (Table 1). This type of resistance requires the health care team to take a multidimensional approach that may include the use of expensive antimicrobial agents and interventional therapies with adjunctive equipment.

Patients can enter acute care facilities predisposed to antimicrobial resistance as the result of an increased risk of colonization or decreased host defense [9]. Indiscriminate antimicrobial use for illnesses of nonbacterial origin (viruses) and

---

* Corresponding author.
E-mail address: massmith@mtsu.edu (M.A. Smith).

0899-5885/07/$ - see front matter © 2007 Elsevier Inc. All rights reserved.
doi:10.1016/j.ccell.2006.10.006

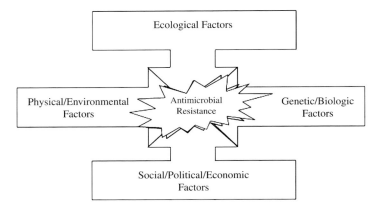

Fig. 1. Converging factors of antimicrobial resistance.

self-diagnosis and treatment with poor-quality drugs or borrowed portions of antimicrobial agents increase the risk of developing antimicrobial-resistant infections [10]. The use of counterfeit antimicrobial agents obtained from Internet-based, non–United States pharmacies is another factor that predisposes the patient to antimicrobial resistance. According to the World Health Organization, the United States represents only 5% of the antimicrobial agents sold worldwide [7]. Approximately 50% of antimicrobial agents are purchased without prescriptions [11]. Many of these are counterfeit or substandard drugs, 51% can carry no active ingredients, 17% contain incorrect ingredients, and 11% contain less than the recommended concentration of active ingredients [7]. The patterns of antimicrobial use noted here,

coupled with the process of antimicrobial natural selection, elevates the potential for resistant strains. Simply put, when antimicrobial agents are administered, bacteria that are more susceptible die. The remaining bacteria are resistant and can pass on this resistant property by replication or conjugation, further complicating the current crisis of antimicrobial resistance [12].

Antimicrobial resistance necessitates the use of further, more expensive antimicrobial agents that quickly increase the economic costs attributable to resistant organisms. These antimicrobial agents can account for up to 30% of a hospital's drug budget [13] and can further compound a patient's in-hospital expenses [14]. According to the US Office of Technology Assessment, the minimum direct hospital costs from five classes of antimicrobial-resistant infections were $1.3 billion in 1992 [8]. Direct costs, however, can be far exceeded by the indirect costs of patient pain and suffering from inadequate antimicrobial treatment [9,11].

Table 1
Types of antimicrobial-resistant organisms

Abbreviation	Antimicrobial-resistant organism
DRSP	Drug-resistant *Streptococcus pneumonia*
ESBLs	Extended-spectrum β-lactamases
MRSA	Methicillin-resistant *Staphylococcus aureus*
MSSA	Methicillin-susceptible *Staphylococcus aureus*
PRSP	Penicillin-resistant *Streptococcus pneumonia*
VISA	Vancomycin-intermediate *Staphylococcus aureus*
VRE	Vancomycin-resistant *Enterococcus*
VRE *faecium*	Vancomycin-resistant *Enterococcus faecium*
VRSA	Vancomycin-resistant *Staphylococcus aureus*

Risk factors for infection

The incidence of underlying disease processes increases with increasing age. Polypharmacy, multiorgan involvement, and compounded disease in the older adult can reduce the ability to combat microorganisms, diminish immune competence, and increase the risk for infection with resistant organisms [8]. In addition, the critical care patient is exposed to numerous risks for infection that augment the emergence of antimicrobial-resistant infections [15]. These risks include, but are not limited to, increased severity of underlying disease processes, multiple invasive procedures, numerous indwelling devices, and extensive use of broad-spectrum antimicrobial agents for prophylaxis and treatment [16]. Because of the nature of critical illness, patients in critical care units undergo more invasive procedures, ranging from endoscopy to bedside surgical intervention, for illnesses such as myocardial infarction and severe burns. Also, indwelling devices are more likely to be used intermittently or for the long term to facilitate patient stabilization and management. Regardless of device, the percentage of infections is higher in patients who have invasive devices than in patients without invasive devices [9]. To improve the quality of care for patients, the Institute of Health Care Improvement launched the 100,000 Lives Campaign. Goals include reducing central line and surgical site infections and ventilator-associated pneumonia. Improvement in the mortality and morbidity associated with these infections would reduce the number of antimicrobial agents used in the critical care unit and thus could reduce the development of antimicrobial resistance.

Patients in critical care units often have multiple disease processes that can predispose them to infection. For example, patients who have chronic lung disease are at an increased risk of developing nosocomial infections [9]. Broad-spectrum antimicrobial agents are often used in an effort to prevent complications that can result from infections in the critical care unit [15]. Although this practice has been common in many critical care units in an attempt to prevent complicated recovery and reduce hospital days, the increased use of antimicrobial agents increases the prevalence of antimicrobial resistance. In fact, use of antimicrobial agents, and in particular "heavy empirical broad-spectrum" antimicrobial agents, may be the most important factor in the progress of antimicrobial resistance [17]. Therefore, this shotgun approach to the treatment of an infection increases the probability that patients will be infected with antimicrobial-resistant microorganisms, resulting in increased morbidity and mortality and increased lengths of stay [18].

Antimicrobial management in critical care

It is commonly agreed that decreasing the amount of antimicrobial agents used will help stabilize antimicrobial resistance. There are additional strategies health care providers can use in vulnerable critical care population.

Guidelines and protocols

Guidelines and protocols can be developed on a local or national level. They can provide evidence-based data on the effectiveness and resistance of specific antimicrobial agents. Although guidelines and protocols can intrude on provider autonomy, they improve patterns of antimicrobial use and resistance [19]. Today, many of these guidelines are available in print format, by personal digital assistant/pocket personal computers, or through Internet access [4]. Professional organizations recommend that local hospitals and communities track and publish antimicrobial surveillance data that include frequency, susceptibility, and resistance information [20]. Reduced costs and significant improvements in quality of care are observed when antimicrobial decisions are based on computer programs factoring epidemiologic information and other relevant patient information [5]. Guidelines, whether local or national, can serve as one option for the individualization of patient management regimens. Computerized and automated systems can identify and minimize antimicrobial adverse drug effects [12,15,21] and prevent inadequate administration [15,22,23]. These systems can reduce problems related to (1) supplying medications to patients with known allergies, (2) adverse antimicrobial events, (3) inaccurate antimicrobial dosing, and (4) costs related to antimicrobial medications [24]. Guidelines and protocols also have been associated with stable antimicrobial susceptibility patterns over time [15]. Appropriate, evidence-based antimicrobial administration may be one component of a multimodal approach to reducing antimicrobial resistance.

Combination antimicrobial therapy

Research is ongoing regarding the ability of combined antimicrobial agents to reduce antimicrobial resistance [25–27]. Some research suggests that resistance to broad-spectrum antimicrobial agents may be reduced over prolonged periods of time by using combination therapy consisting of narrow-spectrum agents [28]. Additionally, combination therapy may be effective as an initial approach to resistant organisms [15]. Research has demonstrated effective responses to certain antimicrobial combinations for nosocomial infections [29], in particular pneumonia [30] and *Mycobacterium tuberculosis* [31]. For example, one study validated a 25% reduction in ceftazidime resistance over 2 years with the use of pipercillin plus an aminoglycocide instead of ceftazidime [32]. In another study, a combination of penicillin G, or ampicillin and an aminoglycocide, provided overall coverage of 94% for empiric antimicrobial treatment in patients who had neutropenic fever [28]. In contrast, other studies report that the advantages of combination therapy remain debatable for treatment of nosocomial pneumonia or septicemias [25,26]. Combination therapy as an approach to reducing bacterial resistance has potential, but additional studies are required to provide adequate support for its use.

Antimicrobial rotation

Rotation or cycling of antimicrobial agents has been presented as a strategy to reduce antimicrobial resistance. This approach entails withdrawing antimicrobial agents by class or individually for a specific period of time and reintroducing the drug later in the antimicrobial treatment regimen in an attempt to reduce the probability of antimicrobial resistance [33,34]. For example, one antimicrobial agent is chosen for a group of critical care patients during a specific period of time, and then a second antimicrobial agent is chosen for another period of time. This process can continue through multiple cycles or rotations. The basic rationale of this approach is that, if the infectious organism develops resistance to the first cycle, it would remain susceptible to the second treatment [35].

Studies have demonstrated that withdrawal of antimicrobial agents by class or individually can potentially restore effectiveness [36,37]. The withdrawal period allows replication of bacteria that subsequently lose resistance to the antimicrobial agent. Other studies, however, indicate that at times cycling may actually lead to increased resistance [38].

At the Minneapolis Veterans Affairs Medical Center, cycling of gentamycin and amikacin proved successful against resistant microbes [39]. Researchers found that the incidence of ventilator-associated pneumonia was reduced by rotation and restricted use of ceftazidime and ciprofloxacin [40]. Rotation of antimicrobial agents shows promise as a strategy to reduce antimicrobial resistance. Optimism should be tempered by the knowledge that further research is needed to identify the most advantageous duration of rotation, number of antimicrobial agents used in the rotation, the types of antimicrobial agents in the protocol, and the order in which they are used [19].

Multidisciplinary team management

The need for antimicrobial agents to treat ongoing and potential bacterial invasion makes antimicrobial resistance an ever-increasing patient care concern. A concerted multidisciplinary effort is required to address antimicrobial resistance in critical care. The categories of health care providers represented on multidisciplinary infection control teams remain diverse. The disciplines represented include microbiologists, pharmacists, infectious disease physicians (or other infectious disease representatives), hospital epidemiologists, nurses, nurse educators, respiratory therapists, and other "infection control personnel." In a survey of 12 countries, the following professions were considered essential members of the multidisciplinary team: infection control physician, nurse/infection control professional, data manager, administrative support, surveillance technician, and epidemiologist. In contrast, others limit the necessary team members to a minimum of a clinical pharmacist and an infectious disease physician and/or clinical microbiologist [41]. Regardless of their composition, these teams can identify areas of concern, assist in the supervision of individuals who have infectious disease, provide information regarding written policies, educate health care providers, and advise administrators [42]. Improved patient care and outcomes and reduced antimicrobial resistance are reported with the use of infectious disease teams [43]. Nurses, in particular critical care nurses, can complement these patient management teams in multiple ways.

Critical care nursing responsibilities

Critical care nurses have specific responsibilities in caring for high-risk, high-acuity patients. Some of these responsibilities include surveillance of antimicrobial resistance patterns in critical care, current knowledge of appropriate antimicrobial use protocols and guidelines, use and enforcement of standard precautions, and specific attention to physiologic defense mechanisms that may increase susceptibility to infection and thus antimicrobial resistance. The Institute of Medicine and the World Health Organization have identified many other interventions, but not all have such a clear association with critical care nurses and patients. Antimicrobial resistance is an important determinant of patient outcome in the critical care units. Through surveillance, application of antimicrobial guidelines, and use of standard precautions (in particular, hand hygiene), critical care nurses can significantly affect transmission of microorganisms.

The multiple responsibilities of critical care nurses continue to grow exponentially. As the number of patients and their acuity increases, the number of nurses decreases. Unfortunately, workload can affect antimicrobial resistance in the critical care unit. Increased patient-to-nurse ratios and reductions in nursing staff increase the rate of infection in ICUs [9,15]. Increased workload can negatively impact compliance with hand-washing procedures in this high-acuity area. Additionally, increased workloads have been equated with prolonged ventilator weaning [44]. The increased ventilator time can predispose the patient to ventilator-associated pneumonia requiring antimicrobial use for treatment.

Hand washing remains the most effective mechanism of nosocomial infection control and prevention [45–47]. Unfortunately, poor compliance with hand washing is common in critical care. It is important that nurses be consistent in the use of hand washing and promote its use by all health care providers and visitors. Critical care nurses also can request the increased use of alcohol-based (at least 60%) hand rubs. These products reduce bacterial counts on hands more effectively than do soap and detergent and in a fraction of the time. The minimal time and effort involved encourages their use. The introduction of these hand rubs has been shown to increase compliance with hand-hygiene recommendations [48,49]. In addition to hand washing, the use of protective devices such as gloves, gowns, and eye shields should be encouraged to further prevent transmission of bacteria.

A common responsibility of nurses is the maintenance of intact skin surfaces. Broken skin surfaces, wounds, and indwelling devices are common in ICUs. These factors put patients at increased risk of infection and thus antimicrobial resistance. Mucous membranes, another external defense mechanism, need protection. Critical care nurses should cleanse and inspect oral mucous membranes routinely, assessing for signs of infection. Brushing teeth and/or rinsing the oral cavity with an antimicrobial agent such as a chlorhexidine solution are components of oral care that can be performed by the critical care nurse. This task has been identified as a positive strategy in reducing ventilator-associated pneumonia [50]. Another example illustrating the importance of intact skin is increased incidence of infection seen in patients who have central lines. As part of the 100,000 Lives Saved campaign, an evidence-based guideline was published that identifies elements that reduce the risk of infections resulting from central lines [51]. Pertinent components of the guideline advocate hand hygiene, barrier precautions, chlorhexidine skin antisepsis, and removal of unnecessary lines. Use of gloves and gowns and adherence to standard precautions are important methods for preventing the spread of microorganisms within a critical care unit. These fundamental nursing responsibilities can deter the introduction of foreign or native flora that can promote infection in an abnormal environment.

Because emergent and life-threatening events are common in the ICU, therapy often begins empirically. It is the responsibility of the physician or advanced practice nurse to prescribe antimicrobial agents for their patients based on current protocols and guidelines. It is the critical care nurse, however, who actually administers the medication. This responsibility provides an ideal opportunity to determine if guidelines and protocols to reduce antimicrobial resistance are followed [52]. Even in high-risk situations that warrant empiric therapy, good antimicrobial stewardship can be supported. Critical care nurses can model this behavior by using data collected regarding the usual organisms seen on the unit, current resistance patterns, and identification of outbreaks with one or more of the locally prevalent organisms. Once culture results are available, empiric antimicrobial therapy can be narrowed appropriately [25].

It is important to track the frequency of resistance at the local level [53]. Surveillance of resistance patterns is another strategy to control the growth of antimicrobial resistance. Additionally, the critical care nurse can ensure that antimicrobial resistance surveillance data guide antimicrobial choices. In some areas, teams actually review requests for antimicrobial agents before the prescription is filled. The use of information technology resources improves the surveillance of antimicrobial resistance and appropriate antimicrobial treatment through data collection, data retrieval, and access to up-to-date guidelines for treatment of organisms commonly seen in critical care [23]. Critical care nurses can make progress in their battle with antimicrobial resistance by using current, evidence-based resources.

Nurses are responsible for the administration of antimicrobial agents on a predetermined schedule. They also must monitor laboratory data for changes that may indicate antimicrobial

Assessment
- Facilitate proper identification of infectious processes by monitoring fluids and secretions (e.g., urine, blood, sputum, etc.).
- Evaluate patient for indications of infectious processes (e.g., vital signs, skin temperature, etc.).

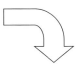

Evaluation
- Monitor patient response to interventions.
- Use response to interventions in research studies to promote patient management through establishment of evidence based nursing guidelines and protocols.

Planning
- Maintain barriers to bacterial invasion (e.g., intact skin, consistent glove and gown use, secure dressings, etc.).
- Incorporate research based interventions.

Implementation
- Administer treatments for identified or potential infectious processes (e.g., administer antibiotics at scheduled times, change dressings as scheduled or as needed, etc.).
- Work to prevent the spread of further microorganism invasion (e.g., proper handwashing, awareness of interventions that predispose patients to microorganisms, staff assignments to prevent potential microorganism spread, etc.).

Fig. 2. Nursing process approach to critical care nursing responsibilities in managing patients who have infectious processes.

effectiveness. It is necessary to ensure that laboratory peak and trough levels be retrieved as ordered for continued patient management. Use of the nursing process can facilitate continued awareness of the cycle of nursing responsibilities when managing the patient with active or potential infectious processes (Fig. 2).

Summary

Patients presenting with active infections or at increased risk for infections pose a significant challenge in critical care nursing. It is important for critical care nurses to use effective antimicrobial strategies in patient management to reduce the potential development of antimicrobial resistance. They should be involved actively in promoting patient management through development of research-based nursing guidelines and protocols.

References

[1] Infectious Disease Society of America (IDSA). Bad bugs, no drugs: an antibiotic discovery stagnates... a public health crisis brews. 2004. Available at: http://www.idsociety.org/pa/IDSA_Paper4_final_web.pdf. Accessed July 5, 2006.

[2] Pronovost PF, Berenholtz SM. Improving sepsis care in the intensive care unit: an evidence-based approach. VHA Research Series. 2004. Available at: http://vhahealthfoundation.org/vhahf/sepsis_icu_execsum.pdf. Accessed June 18, 2006.

[3] Kopp FJ, Nix DE, Armstrong EP. Clinical and economic analysis of methicillin-susceptible and -resistant Staphylococcus aureus infections. Ann Pharmacother 2004;38:1377–82.

[4] Plonczynski DJ, Plonczynski KJ. Antibiotic resistance: the impact on care of hospitalized patients. Medsurg Nurs 2005;14:160–6.

[5] Sing N, Yu VL. Rational empiric antibiotic prescription in the ICU: clinical research is mandatory. Chest 2000;117:1496–9.

[6] Kollef MH, Fraser VJ. Antibiotic resistance in the intensive care unit. Ann Intern Med 2001;134:298–314.

[7] World Health Organization. Factors contributing to resistance. Infection disease report; 2000. Available at: http://www.who.int/infectious-disease-report/2000/ch3.htm. Accessed June 28, 2006.

[8] Emerging trends in antibiotic resistance: strategies for appropriate antibiotic use. Formulary 2005; 40(Suppl 1):S3–15.

[9] Vincent JL. Nosocomial infections in adult intensive-care units. Lancet 2003;361:2068–77.

[10] Centers for Disease Control and Prevention. Department of Health and Human Services. Available at: http://www.cdc.gov. Accessed June 19, 2006.

[11] Cars O, Nordberg P. Antibiotic resistance—the faceless threat. The International Journal of Risk & Safety in Medicine 2005;17:103–10.

[12] Workman ML. The cellular basis of bacterial infection. Crit Care Nurs Clin North Am 2003;15(1): 1–11.

[13] DeLisle S, Perl TM. Antimicrobial management measures to limit resistance: a process-based conceptual framework. Crit Care Med 2001;29(4):N121–7.

[14] Classen DC, Pestonik SL, Evans RS, et al. Adverse drug events in hospitalized patients. Excess length of stay, extra costs, and attributable mortality. JAMA 1997;277:301–6.

[15] Kollef MH. Optimizing antibiotic therapy in the intensive care unit setting. Crit Care 2001;5:189–95.

[16] Puzniak LA, Mayfield J, Leet T, et al. Acquisition of vancomycin-resistant enterococci during scheduled antimicrobial rotation in an intensive care unit. Clin Infect Dis 2001;33:151–7.

[17] Broadhead JM, Parra DS, Skelton PA. Emerging multiresistant organisms in the ICU: epidemiology, risk factors, surveillance, and prevention. Crit Care Nurs Q 2001;24:20–9.

[18] Ibrahim EH, Ward S, Sherman G, et al. A comparative analysis of patients with early-onset versus late-onset nosocomial pneumonia (NP) in the ICU setting. Chest 2000;117:1434–42.

[19] Askari R, Sawyer RG. New antibacterial administration treatment strategies. Surg Infect 2005; 6(Suppl 2):s-83–s-95.

[20] Strausbaugh LJ, Siegel JD, Weinstein RA. Preventing transmission of multidrug-resistant bacteria in health care settings: a tale of 2 guidelines. Clin Infect Dis 2006;42(6):828–35.

[21] Pestotnik SL, Classen DC, Evans RS, et al. Prospective surveillance of imipenem/cilastin use and associated seizures using a hospital information system. Ann Pharmacother 1993;27:497–501.

[22] Evans RS, Classes DC, Pestotnik SL, et al. Improving empiric antibiotic selection using computer decision support. Arch Intern Med 1994;154:878–84.

[23] Drew RH, Kawamoto K, Adams MB. Information technology for optimizing the management of infectious diseases. Am J Health Syst Pharm 2006;63(10): 957–65.

[24] Evans RS, Pestotnik SL, Classes DC, et al. A computer assisted management program for antibiotic and other antiinfective agents. N Engl J Med 1998; 338:232–8.

[25] Bergogne-Berezin E. Treatment and prevention of nosocomial pneumonia. Chest 1999;108:26S–34S.

[26] Siegman-Igra Y, Ravona R, Primerman H, et al. Pseudomonas aeruginosa bacteremia: an analysis of 123 episodes, with particular emphasis on the effect of antibiotic therapy. Int J Infect Dis 1998;2: 211–5.

[27] Fish DN, Ohlinger MJ. Antimicrobial resistance: factors and outcomes. Crit Care Clin 2006;22: 291–311.

[28] Kristensen B, Smedeggard HH, Pedersen HM, et al. Antibiotic resistance patterns among blood culture isolates in a Danish county 1981–1995. J Med Microbiol 1999;48:67–71.

[29] Orbitsch MD, Fish DN, MacLaren R, et al. Nosocomial infections due to multidrug-resistant Pseudomonas aeruginosa: epidemiology and treatment options. Pharmacotherapy 2005;25(10):1353–64.

[30] Trouillet JL, Chastre J, Vuagnat A, et al. Ventilator-assisted pneumonia caused by potentially drug-resistant bacteria. Am J Respir Crit Care Med 1998;157: 531–9.

[31] McGowen JE Jr, Gerding DN. Does antibiotic restriction prevent resistance? New Horiz 1996;4: 370–6.

[32] Mebis J, Goossens H, Bruyneel P, et al. Decreasing antibiotic resistance of Enterobacteriaceae by introducing a new antibiotic combination therapy for neutropenic fever patients. Leukemia 1998;12: 1627–9.

[33] Niederman MS. Is "crop rotation" of antibiotics the solution to a "resistant" problem in the ICU? Am J Respir Crit Care Med 1997;156:1029–31.

[34] Masterton RG. Antibiotic cycling: more than it might seem? J Antimicrob Chemother 2005;55: 1–5.

[35] Pechere JC. Commentary: rotating antibiotics in the intensive care unit: feasible, apparently beneficial, but questions remain. Crit Care 2002;6:9–10.

[36] Climo MW, Israel DS, Wong ES, et al. Hospital-wide restriction of clindamycin effect on the incidence of *Clostridium difficile*-associated diarrhea and cost. Ann Intern Med 1998;128:989–95.

[37] Quale J, Landman D, Saurina G, et al. Manipulation of a hospital antimicrobial formulary to control an outbreak of vancomycin-resistant enterococci. Clin Infect Dis 1996;23:1020–5.

[38] Fishman N. Antimicrobial stewardship. Am J Med 2006;119(Suppl 6A):S53–61 Available at: EBSCOhost Research database online. Accessed July 19, 2006.

[39] Gerding DN, Larson TA, Hughes RA, et al. Aminoglycoside resistance and aminoglycoside usage: ten years of experience in one hospital. Antimicrob Agents Chemother 1991;35:1284–90.

[40] Gruson D, Hibert G, Vargas F, et al. Rotation and restricted use of antibiotics in a medical intensive care unit: impact on the incidence of ventilator associated pneumonia caused by antibiotic-resistant gram-negative bacteria. Am J Respir Crit Care Med 2000;162:837–43.

[41] Voss A, Allerberger F, Bouza E, et al. The training curriculum in hospital infection control. Clin Microbiol Infect 2005;11(Suppl 1):33–5.

[42] Gordts B. Models for the organization of hospital infection control and prevention programmes. Clin Microbiol Infect 2005;11(Suppl 1):19–23.

[43] Weeks C, Jones G, Wyllie S. Cost and health care benefits of an antimicrobial management programme. Hosp Pharm 2006;13:179–82. Available at: http://www.pjonline.com/pdf/hp/200605/hp_200605_antimicrobial.pdf. Accessed June 19, 2006.

[44] Thoren JB, Kaelin RM, Jolliet P, et al. Influence of the quality of nursing on the duration of weaning from mechanical ventilation in patients with chronic obstructive pulmonary disease. Crit Care Med 1995; 23:1807–15.

[45] Jarvis WR. Handwashing–the Semmelweis lesson forgotten? Lancet 1994;344:1311–2.

[46] Goldmann D, Larson E. Hand-washing and nosocomial infections [editorial]. Lancet 1992;327: 120–2.

[47] Doebbeling BN, Stanley GI, Sheetz CT, et al. Comparative efficacy of alternate hand-washing agents in reducing nosocomial infections in intensive care units. N Engl J Med 1992;327:88–93.

[48] Fry DA, Burger TL. Hand hygiene compliance: step up, reach out. Nurs Manage 2006;37(3):40–3.

[49] LAM BC, Lee JL, Lau YL. Hand hygiene practices in a neonatal intensive care unit: a multimodal intervention and impact on nosocomial infection. Pediatrics 2004;114:565–71.

[50] O'keefe-McCarthy S. Evidence-based nursing strategies to prevent ventilator-acquired pneumonia. Dynamics 2006;17(1):8–11.

[51] Institute for Healthcare Improvement. Getting started kit: preventing central line infections. Available at: http://ihi.org/NR/rdonlyres/BF4CC102-C564-4436-AC3A-0C57B1202872/0/CentralLinesHowtoGuide-FINAL720.pdf. Accessed July 23, 2006.

[52] Bissett L. Reducing the risk of acquiring antimicrobial-resistant bacteria. Br J Nurs 2006;15:68–71.

[53] Farner SM. Use of local community hospital data for surveillance of antimicrobial resistance. Infect Control Hosp Epidemiol 2006;27(3):299–301.

ELSEVIER
SAUNDERS

Crit Care Nurs Clin N Am 19 (2007) 61–68

CRITICAL CARE
NURSING CLINICS
OF NORTH AMERICA

Methicillin-Resistant *Staphylococcus aureus* in Critical Care Areas

John Travis Dunlap, MSN, APRN, BC

Adult Nurse Practitioner Program, Vanderbilt University School of Nursing, 461, 21st Avenue South, 367 Frist Hall, Nashville, TN 37240, USA

Epidemic, and now more recently endemic, methicillin-resistant *Staphylococcus aureus* (MRSA) infections have been an ever-increasing reality in the modern hospital environment since it was first isolated in 1961 [1]. According to a recent study by Cosgrove and colleagues [2], MRSA is now the isolated organism in 55% of ICU nosocomial infections in the United States, and this number will continue to increase for the near future. This increase becomes more concerning because MRSA infections have been shown to have a higher morbidity and mortality than a methicillin-sensitive S*taphylococcus aureus* (MSSA) infection. Cosgrove and colleagues [3] performed a meta-analysis that identified 31 cohort studies that contained data regarding the mortality associated with both MSSA and MRSA bacteremia. Seven of these studies found significantly higher mortality rates associated with MRSA bacteremia, whereas the remaining studies found no difference in mortality rates ($P < .001$). It is an understatement to say MRSA infections play a significant role in impacting patient care in critical care areas especially considering these patients are typically already compromised by other disease sequelae and/or are immunocompromised as well. Consequently a review of current literature and an overview of MRSA in the critical care setting is considered an appropriate and prudent measure in improving patient care as it relates to MRSA infections.

Evolution of *Staphylococcus aureus* to methicillin-resistant *Staphylococcus aureus*

Staphylococcus aureus (*S aureus*) belongs to the Micrococcaceae family and are gram-positive cocci; each individual organism is approximately one micrometer in diameter that normally coalesces with other *S aureus* nearby into grape-like clusters. *S aureus* is distinguished from other staphylococcal varieties by the gold pigmentation of its colonies (*aureus* is Latin for "golden"), production of the enzyme coagulase, and other subtle differences that require advanced genetic testing such as pulsed-field gel electrophoresis to be elicited [4]. *S aureus* is pathogenic and was identified as a causative agent in diseases as early as the 1880s. *S aureus* is a very adaptable organism, and this was demonstrated with the advent of mass-produced penicillin to fight bacterial infections starting in the early 1940s. By 1944, studies were being published describing penicillinase-producing strains of *S aureus* that were the first indications of *S aureus* resistance [5]. By 1950, 40% of hospital *S aureus* isolates were penicillin-resistant; in 1960, this had risen to 80%, and now the prevalence of penicillin resistance in *S aureus* is well in excess of 90% [6]. Methicillin, a semisynthetic penicillinase-resistant penicillin, was introduced in 1959 to treat penicillin-resistant *S aureus* infections, but in only 2 years there were reports that methicillin resistant *S aureus* had been isolated in the United Kingdom and now accounts for 55% of ICU nosocomial infections in the United States [1,2].

Methicillin resistance is conferred by the methicillin-resistant gene (*mecA*) that encodes for production of a penicillin-binding protein not present in methicillin-susceptible strains of *S aureus*.

E-mail address: travis.dunlap@vanderbilt.edu

doi:10.1016/j.ccell.2006.10.010

ccnursing.theclinics.com

Modern polymerase chain reaction analysis is now the benchmark for confirming if a strain of S aureus is MRSA by detecting the presence of the mecA gene [1]. One noteworthy aspect of the mecA gene is its location on a mobile genetic element: the staphylococcal chromosome cassette mec (SCCmec). There are at least five forms of the SCCmec known as types I, II, III, IV, and, more recently, V. Hospital-associated MRSA infections are mainly of types I, II and III, whereas community-associated MRSA are type IV. Typically these mobile genetic elements allow microorganisms to acquire the necessary genes for developing antibiotic resistance by spontaneous genetic mutation, but this has only been the case regarding S aureus a few times [5]. Hence, the global emergence of MRSA is not from the constant mutation of MSSA bacteria but the distribution of a few MRSA clones around the world [7]. This detail highlights the importance of minimizing the transmission of MRSA to minimize the number of MRSA outbreaks that are commonly experienced in acute care settings.

Methicillin-resistant Staphylococcus aureus epidemiology

S aureus is typically an innocuous passenger in the human body that may colonize the face, hands, axilla, groin, and most commonly, the anterior nares. A recent study of 9929 persons at least 1 year of age participating in the National Health and Nutrition Examination Survey showed that 2964 people were colonized with S aureus in the anterior nares [8]. The authors estimated the weighted S aureus colonization prevalence in the United States population to be 32.4% (95% confidence interval (CI), 30.7%–34.1%) or 89.4 million persons (95% CI, 84.8–94.1 million persons). The study also determined that 0.8% (95% CI, 0.4%–1.4%) or 2.3 million persons (95% CI, 1.2–3.8 million) are colonized with MRSA. This prevalence demonstrates that S aureus is an ecologically successful organism that adapts well to its environment. In fact a recent study demonstrates the number of MRSA-colonized persons is continuing to increase at a vigorous rate. Investigators in Nashville, Tennessee, compared the frequency of community-associated MRSA nasal colonization in 2001 to more recent data in 2004 [9]. In 2001, specimens were gathered from the anterior nares of 500 children using nasal swabs, and 4 children (0.8%) were found to be carriers for MRSA. In 2004, using the same techniques, 500 children

were tested, and 46 children (9.2%) were colonized with MRSA, a greater than 10-fold increase in 3 years ($P < .001$).

Risk factors for colonization and infection

Concern should be raised regarding the presence of MRSA colonization because a significant risk factor for MRSA infections is a person already colonized with S aureus [8,10,11]. In fact, Merrer and colleagues [11] demonstrated that above a 30% colonization pressure (the number of MRSA carrier patient days divided by the total number of patient days), the risk of acquiring an MRSA infection was almost 5 times higher ($P < .001$).

At least one prospective cohort study narrowed the risk factors to a specific patient population of surgical intensive care patients that identified risk factors for MRSA colonization on admission and acquisition of MRSA while on the surgical ICU. Warren and colleagues [10] performed active surveillance with nasal cultures on 1469 patients of the 1494 admitted (98%) over a 15-month period and performed risk factor analysis on 775 patients (53%) who stayed in the surgical ICU for greater than 48 hours. Factors independently associated with MRSA colonization on admission were: one or more admissions to the study hospital in the past year, a hospital length of stay of 5 days or more before admission to the surgical ICU, chronic obstructive pulmonary disease, diabetes mellitus, and isolation of MRSA in the past 6 months [10]. This last risk factor was the most significant and demonstrated that patients who have a history of MRSA colonization in the previous 6 months were 8 times more likely to be colonized with MRSA on admission to the surgical ICU [10]. Risk factors associated for becoming colonized with MRSA in the surgical ICU included: tracheostomy in the ICU; development of a decubitus ulcer while in the ICU; and enteral nutrition by way of nasoenteric tube, percutaneous feeding tube, or both nasoenteric and percutaneous tube [10]. Tube feeding by way of a percutaneous tube alone did not significantly elevate the risk of MRSA acquisition, which suggests that the route was the risk factor rather than tube feeding solution itself [10].

All bacterial infections occur as a result of a breakdown in either the skin or mucosal membranes that allow the organism, in this case MRSA, means of access to underlying tissues and possibly the vascular system as well. The resulting infection's severity will be determined by several factors including the nutritional status of the infected person, the status of their immune system, genetic predisposition, and virulence of MRSA among others [7]. As with most infectious diseases, identification of risk factors may help to identify an MRSA infection earlier in its course, reduce or remove potential reservoirs, and influence subsequent modalities of treatment. Multiple causes for the incidence of general MRSA infections have been put forward including colonization pressure as well as recent hospitalization or surgery, residing in a long-term–care facility, any type of indwelling catheter, enteral feedings, prior macrolide use and levofloxacin antibiotic usage, an immunocompromised state, or intravenous drug use [12–14].

Methicillin-resistant *Staphylococcus aureus* virulence and infections

Not only does the chromosome of *S aureus* encode methicillin resistance but it also determines what toxins the organism will be able to produce during an infection, thus affecting how virulent the organism will be to any potential host. Nearly all strains of staphylococci convert host tissue to nutrients by way of enzymes such as hemolysins, nucleases, proteases, lipases, hyaluronidase, and collagenase. Although their role in pathogenesis is not fully understood, the end result is destruction of host tissues. These bacterial enzymes make possible the spread of infection to adjoining tissues [4,15] and contribute to the heterogeneity of *S aureus* infections, including toxic shock syndrome, bacteremia, endocarditis, metastatic infections, and sepsis [4].

S aureus produces numerous toxins that are classified according to their mechanism of action and are found in varying percentages in different *S aureus* isolates. The four most common exotoxins are reviewed: staphylococcal enterotoxins, toxic shock syndrome toxin-1, exfoliative toxins, and Panton–Valentine leukocidin. All these toxins are known to be pyrogenic (fever producing), and they also function as superantigens [16,17]. Superantigens bind to major histocompatability complexes outside of the normal binding site and cause considerable T-cell proliferation leading to massive cytokine release and subsequent shock. Kim and colleagues [16] noted that almost 96% of the MRSA SCCmec II (nosocomial) strains carried staphylococcal toxin genes compared with 74.4% of SCCmec III (also nosocomial) strains and 68.8% of SCCmec IV (community-associated MRSA) strains. In contrast, only 53.8% of MSSA

strains produced these toxins. MRSA strains may be more virulent than MSSA strains.

One group of toxins produced by *S aureus* that contains at least nine major types is the staphylococcal enterotoxins, most notable for their role in staphylococcal food poisoning. Because of its high tolerance to heat and relatively high resistance to proteolysis, *S aureus* can endure both the heating of food and digestion in the stomach, and ingestion of staphylococcal enterotoxins-containing food products induces vomiting that is often accompanied by gastroenteritis [18].

Toxic shock syndrome toxin-1 is another toxin secreted by some *S aureus* isolates that is structurally similar to the staphylococcal enterotoxins group. Toxic shock syndrome toxin-1 is encoded by the *tst* gene and is the major virulence factor in toxic shock syndrome, staphylococcal scarlet fever, and neonatal toxic shock-like exanthematous diseases. Toxic shock syndrome is a disease characterized by rapid onset of fever, hypotension, erythematous rash, and mucosal hyperemia, followed by desquamation and multiorgan involvement. Toxic shock syndrome was initially linked to the introduction of superabsorbent tampon use during menstruation until education campaigns warned of the risks and now nonmenstruation-associated toxic shock syndrome is more prevalent and more lethal, occurring secondary to local *S aureus* infection [19].

There are two known exfoliative toxin serotypes known as epidermolytic toxins A and B (ETA and ETB) that are expressed by genes *eta* and *etb*, respectively. ETA and ETB are responsible for causing skin erythema and separation as seen in staphylococcal scalded-skin syndrome [20]. Panton–Valentine leukocidin toxin will also be included here despite the fact that Panton–Valentine leukocidin is typically associated with community-associated MRSA, which is identified by genetic testing as having SCCmec IV or V genetic element [21]. Panton–Valentine leukocidin is a leukocytolitic toxin that causes leukocyte destruction, tissue necrosis, and is epidemiologically associated with severe cutaneous infections and necrotizing pneumonia [15].

Methicillin-resistant *Staphylococcus aureus* morbidity and mortality outcomes

Along with Cosgrove and colleagues [3], there are numerous studies that have looked at morbidity as well as mortality of MRSA infections as compared with MSSA infections; three are discussed here [22–24]. Blott and colleagues [22] showed that patients who had MRSA bacteremia had more acute renal failure and hemodynamic instability than patients who had MSSA bacteremia as well as a longer ICU stay and ventilator dependency. Patients who had MRSA bacteremia also had a higher 30-day mortality rate and in-hospital mortality rate overall. A study by pharmacists at the University of Arizona at Tucson showed patients who had MRSA infections had a trend toward longer hospital length of stay and longer antibiotic-related length of stay as well as more frequent antibiotic treatment failure [23]. Finally, a more recent study looked at patients 18 or over admitted to two hospitals over a 7-year period that included 250,000 patients. The overall mortality 30 days after staphylococcal bacteremia was 29%; however, the death rate from MRSA (34%) was higher than that for MSSA (27%) [24]. This emphasizes the need for better infection control, surveillance measures, and effective medical therapy in our health care facilities.

Infection control

As the arsenal of successful antibiotic therapies shrinks, reducing MRSA colonization and infections through infection control and other methods needs to take on a more prominent role in our modern hospitals. In 2000, as the rate of MRSA and vancomycin-resistant *enterococcus* continued to increase, the Society for Healthcare Epidemiology of America (SHEA) board of directors appointed a taskforce to compose an evidence-based guideline on preventing nosocomial transmission of pathogens with a focus on vancomycin-resistant *enterococcus* and MRSA [7]. The guidelines were released in 2003 and observed, "There have been no published reports of MRSA being eradicated through antibiotic control programs alone. On the other hand, interventions leading to eradication from individual nursing units or entire hospitals have been based primarily on preventing person-to-person spread with less emphasis on antibiotic control" [7]. There are multiple studies that demonstrate MRSA can be controlled through thorough infection control practices [25–27]. Halting the spread of MRSA and actually diminishing its prevalence is a reality in certain regions of the world, including the northern European countries of the Netherlands, Denmark, Sweden, and Finland, where the prevalence of MRSA isolates as a total

of all *S aureus* isolates is less than 1% as compared with greater than 40% in southern and western Europe including Germany and England [25].

It is impossible to discuss infection control without mentioning hand hygiene. Several studies have demonstrated how contaminated the health care environment is, including not only the hospital patient rooms but also medical equipment such as computers [28–30]. French and colleagues [29] found that 74% of rooms previously occupied by MRSA-colonized or infected patients were contaminated with MRSA before standard cleaning per established guidelines, and that 66% of the rooms still yielded MRSA after standard cleaning. The Centers of Disease Control in Prevention has recommended hand washing after each and every patient contact as part of standard precautions since 1996 [31], but unfortunately compliance of this regulation has been unacceptably low [32,33]. However, Boyce and Pittet [33] and Gordin and colleagues [34] have observed that, with the advent of alcohol-based hand rubs and recent improvements in the understanding of the epidemiology of hand hygiene compliance, the incidence of nosocomial infections can be reduced. The SHEA guidelines state that health care workers should use antiseptic-containing preparations to decontaminate their hands before and after all patient contact even if clean and/or sterile gloves are worn [7,33]. This includes any patient contact such as taking a pulse or lifting them up in bed or any coming into contact with inanimate objects that has touched the patient such as a blood pressure cuff or bedside table [7,33].

Active surveillance is another recommendation of the SHEA task force guidelines and has been credited for the low MRSA prevalence of northern European countries because of "search and destroy" policies [7,25,26]. Still there is controversy as to what extent these guidelines should be implemented. One concern with active surveillance may be the cost associated with implementing such programs because of the equipment and laboratories required to screen patients for MRSA. A study by Clancy and colleagues [35] took costs into account and looked at the cost-effectiveness of implementing an active surveillance system. In the study, all patients 18 years or older admitted or transferred to a medical ICU or surgical ICU at the study hospital had a baseline nasal swab performed, and at least one every week there after as long as they stayed in the medical ICU or surgical ICU. The patients who tested positive for MRSA were placed on contact isolation that included a private room and required every person entering to wear gowns and gloves [35]. The study showed a statistically significant decrease in the rate of all MRSA infections despite an increase in the number of community-associated MRSA-based infections that were admitted to other units in the hospital [35]. The program averted approximately 2.5 MRSA infections per month in both units, avoiding $19,714 in excess cost despite the cost of supplies needed for contact isolation [35]. Some institutions may not be able to provide the resources needed to test every patient admitted or transferred to a unit. Therefore, Warren and colleagues [10] looked at screening patients at high risk and those with known risk factors for MRSA colonization. They found that screening based on significant risk factors would identify 89% of MRSA-colonized patients and would decrease the total number of admission surveillance cultures by 42% [10]. The SHEA guidelines suggest that effective control of MRSA that includes an active surveillance system would result in cost savings between $20,062 and $462,067 annually and would prevent 8 to 41 MRSA infections [7]. The SHEA guidelines recommend implementing an active surveillance program that screen patients at high risk for carriage on admission and periodically thereafter [7].

Another recommendation of the SHEA task force is barrier precautions, or contact isolation, for patients known or suspected to be colonized or infected with MRSA [7]. The guidelines suggest that gloves and masks should always be worn to enter the room and that gowns should always be worn except when there is no direct contact with the patient or environmental surfaces [7]. One study that demonstrated the success of barrier precautions discovered that patients who are colonized or infected with MRSA but do not have barrier precautions in place are 16 times more likely to spread MRSA to health care workers and other patients than patients who are under contact isolation [36].

The final SHEA task force guideline to be discussed is the decolonization or suppression of colonized patients. A significant colonization pressure increases the risk of acquiring a MRSA infection [11]. Therefore, one possible approach to preventing MRSA infections would be to decolonize patients and health care workers identified as being carriers. One analysis demonstrating the impact of nasal MRSA colonization compared *S aureus* strains isolated from the anterior nares to those isolated in the blood of patients who have *S aureus* bacteremia using pulsed-field gel electrophoresis. This study found that at least 50% of patients who have *S aureus* bacteremia were first colonized in the anterior nares by an identical strain [37]. A commonly used treatment for decolonization of the anterior nares is intranasal mupirocin ointment applied two to three times daily and a shower with 4% chlorhexidine once daily for 5 days for decolonization of the groin, axilla, face, and hands [38]. The SHEA task force guidelines clarified that widespread prolonged use should be avoided because this has been associated with the evolution and spread of antibiotic resistant strains [7]. Any decolonization program should limit use to selected populations including patients and health care workers colonized with MRSA, and the program should incorporate routine susceptibility testing to evaluate its effectiveness [7].

There is, however, conflicting evidence regarding the success of such active surveillance, patient isolation as it relates to cohorting of care (which was not offered as an infection control method in the SHEA guidelines [7]), and contact isolation; there is also a lack of randomized control trials evaluating these techniques [39,40]. For instance, Loveday and colleagues [39] looked at evidence for interventions for prevention and control of MRSA over an 8-year timeframe and concluded that, "There is currently insufficient high-quality evidence for infection prevention and control interventions in the fields identified for this review." This matches the analysis of another review by Cooper and colleagues [40] that states, "No well-designed studies exist that allow the role of isolation measures alone to be assessed." Loveday and colleagues [39] and Cooper and colleagues [40] concur that national guidelines should continue to be applied until more reliable research establishes another course of action.

Perceptions and culture change

Infection control policies exist and yet interventions, such as hand washing, have low compliance rates despite the fact that there is strong evidence to show they reduce MRSA infection rates [7,31,33]. A small qualitative study set out to examine the extent to which staff nurses feel that MRSA is out of control and that any attempt, by them, to control it is unnecessary [41]. Fifteen nurses with at least 5 years of experience were randomly interviewed at a university teaching hospital [41]. The study is small and may not translate to other settings, but some of the perceptions support the poor compliance rates found in other studies [32,33]. These nurses considered themselves to be team leaders and role models, yet 60% of the participants believed that MRSA is out of control, and asked, "Why should they worry about it?" Nearly 80% admitted that prescribed mupirocin doses were frequently missed [41]. The author felt that the cause for the apathy and nonadherence were related to poor subject knowledge and that this culture was perpetuated to junior staff by the more senior nurses [41]. Another theme was frustration with issues of understaffing where screening and contact precautions were viewed as a "chore," and frustration with physicians who did not follow infection control precautions [41]. Overall, the author observed that there were gaps in education and compliance and that nursing management should initiate and support actions to improve the culture [41].

Culture change that enables health care workers to be more compliant and to improve patient outcomes is an appropriate response to these perceptions. One regional hospital observed a similar culture and was motivated to initiate and implement a 3-year program that had a goal of improving hand hygiene compliance, to introduce better cleaning of shared ward equipment, and to offer MRSA decolonization to a targeted group of known colonized patients on readmission to specific units [42]. Over the 3 years, interventions, such as better access to alcohol-based hand cleaners and alcohol impregnated wipes for shared equipment, were made available. In addition, an aggressive culture change program that included an advertising consultant to fully disseminate their desired goal to the staff [42] was instituted. Hand hygiene compliance doubled from 21% to 42% and was maintained for a year. The MRSA colonization rate in patients decreased from 1507 patients preintervention to 697 at 12 months postintervention but there was no statistically significant change in health care worker colonization. Finally there was a statistically significant decrease in MRSA infections at the end of the 3-year program [42]. Sufficient culture change is an attainable goal that results in lower rates of MRSA infections.

Summary

In recent years the mainstay of treatment for hospital-associated MRSA infections has been vancomycin, but now vancomycin intermediate *S aureus* strains are beginning to emerge. Complete vancomycin resistant *S aureus* can develop, possessing the same *vanA* gene as vancomycin-resistant enterococcus. Four such isolates have been reported, three of which have been in the United States [43]. There are new antibiotics being developed, but there is always a risk of resistance developing. There are some promising new ideas such as staphylococcal conjugate vaccines that reduce the rates of *S aureus* bacteremia for up to 10 months postimmunization in patients who have end stage renal disease receiving hemodialysis, but studies are ongoing [44]. With all the uncertainty surrounding treatment, at least one medium has remained consistent and effective if used properly—infection control. But this requires complete support of all health care workers and hospital administration from the chief medical officer to doctors and nurses to environmental services personnel to take ownership of an effective infection control program.

Who will advocate for more stringent infection control policies and for the equipment to successfully carry them out? Who will take the lead by ensuring implementation of infection control policies on a unit is effective? Who will hold themselves and other health care workers including physicians accountable to comply with these infection control policies every time they enter a patient's room? Nurses are on the front lines in the battle against antibiotic-resistant nosocomial infections such as MRSA, and we should not be apathetic or feel we are helpless. It is our duty as patient advocates not to take a spectator role but to answer these questions: "I will."

Acknowledgments

This author is grateful for the assistance, advice, and friendship of Dr. C. Buddy Creech 2nd.

References

[1] Enright MC, Robinson DA, Randle G, et al. The evolutionary history of methicillin-resistant *Staphylococcus aureus* (MRSA). Proc Natl Acad Sci USA 2002;99:7687–92.
[2] Cosgrove SE, Qi Y, Kaye KS. The impact of methicillin resistance in *Staphylococcus aureus* bacteremia on patient outcomes: mortality, length of stay, and hospital charges. Infect Control Hosp Epidemiol 2005;26:166–74.
[3] Cosgrove SE, Sakoulas G, Perencevich EN, et al. Comparison of mortality associated with methicillin-resistant and methicillin-susceptible *Staphylococcus aureus* bacteremia: a meta-analysis. Clin Infect Dis 2003;36:53–9.

[4] Lowy FD. *Staphylococcus aureus* infections. N Engl J Med 1998;339:520–32.

[5] Rolinson GN. A discussion on penicillin and related antibiotics—past, present and future. Proc R Soc Lond B Biol Sci 1971;179:403–10.

[6] Chambers HF. The changing epidemiology of *Staphylococcus aureus*. Emerg Infect Dis 2001;7: 178–82.

[7] Muto CA, Jernigan JA, Ostrowsky BE, et al. SHEA guideline for preventing nosocomial transmission of multidrug – resistant strains of *Staphylococcus aureus* and *Enterococcus*. Infect Control Hosp Epidemiol 2003;24:639–41.

[8] Kuehnert MJ, Kruszon-Moran D, Hill H, et al. Prevalence of *Staphylococcus aureus* nasal colonization in the United States, 2001–2002. J Infect Dis 2006;193:172–9.

[9] Creech CB 2nd, Kernodle DS, Alsentzer A, et al. Increasing rates of nasal carriage of methicillin-resistant *Staphylococcus aureus* in healthy children. Pediatr Infect Dis J 2005;24:617–21.

[10] Warren DK, Guth RM, Coopersmith CM, et al. Epidemiology of methicillin – resistant *Staphylococcus aureus* colonization in a surgical intensive care unit. Infect Control Hosp Epidemiol 2006;27:1032–40.

[11] Merrer J, Santoli F, Appere de Vecchi C, et al. "Colonization pressure" and risk of acquisition of methicillin-resistant Staphylococcus aureus in a medical intensive care unit. Infect Control Hosp Epidemiol 2000;21:718–23.

[12] Federal Bureau of Prisons—Clinical Practice Guidelines. Management of methicillin – resistant *Staphylococcus aureus* (MRSA) infections. Available at: http://www.bop.gov/news/PDFs/mrsa.pdf. 2005. Accessed October 10, 2006.

[13] Graffunder EM, Venezia RA. Risk factors associated with nosocomial methicillin-resistant *Staphylococcus aureus* (MRSA) infection including previous use of antimicrobials. J Antimicrob Chemother 2002; 49:999–1005.

[14] Huang SS, Platt R. Risk of methicillin – resistant *Staphylococcus aureus* infection after previous infection or colonization. Clin Infect Dis 2003;36:281–5.

[15] Boubaker K, Diebold P, Blank, et al. Panton-valentine leukocidin and staphylococcal skin infections in schoolchildren. Emerg Infect Dis 2004;10:121–4.

[16] Kim JS, Song W, Kim HS, et al. Association between the methicillin resistance of clinical isolates of *Staphylococcus aureus*, their staphylococcal cassette chromosome mec (SCCmec) subtype classification, and their toxin gene profiles. Diagn Microbiol Infect Dis Jul 17, 2006 [Epub ahead of print].

[17] Becker K, Friedrich AW, Lubritz G. Prevalence of genes encoding pyrogenic toxin superantigens and exfoliative toxins among strains of *Staphylococcus aureus* isolated from blood and nasal specimens. J Clin Microbiol 2003;41:1434–9.

[18] Bania J, Dabrowska A, Korzekwa K, et al. The profiles of enterotoxin genes in *Staphylococcus aureus* from nasal carriers. Lett Appl Microbiol 2006; 42(4):315–20.

[19] Durand G, Bes M, Meugnier H, et al. Detection of new methicillin – resistant *Staphylococcus aureus* clones containing the toxic shock syndrome toxin 1 gene responsible for hospital – and community – acquired infections in France. J Clin Microbiol 2006;44:847–53.

[20] Becker K, Roth R, Peters G. Rapid and specific detection of toxigenic *Staphylococcus aureus*: use of two multiplex PCR enzyme immunoassays for amplification and hybridization of staphylococcal enterotoxin genes, exfoliative toxin genes, and toxic shock syndrome toxin 1 gene. J Clin Microbiol 1998;36:2548–53.

[21] Davis SL, Rybak MJ, Amjad M, et al. Characteristics of patients with healthcare-associated infection due to SCCmec Type IV methicillin-resistant *Staphylococcus aureus*. Infect Control Hosp Epidemiol 2006;27:1025–31.

[22] Blot SI, Vandewoude KH, Hoste EA, et al. Outcome and attributable mortality in critically ill patients with bacteremia involving methicillin-susceptible and methicillin-resistant *Staphylococcus aureus*. Arch Intern Med 2002;162:2229–35.

[23] Kopp BJ, Nix DE, Armstrong EP. Clinical and economic analysis of methicillin-susceptible and -resistant *Staphylococcus aureus* infections. Ann Pharmacother 2004;38:1377–82.

[24] Wyllie DH, Crook DW, Peto TE. Mortality after *Staphylococcus aureus* bacteraemia in two hospitals in Oxfordshire, 1997–2003: cohort study. BMJ 2006; 333(7562):281 [Epub 2006, Jun 23]. Available at: http://bmj.bmjjournals.com/cgi/reprint/333/7562/ 281. Accessed October 13, 2006.

[25] Tiemersma EW, Bronzwaer SL, Lyytikainen O, et al. European antimicrobial resistance surveillance system participants. Methicillin-resistant *Staphylococcus aureus* in Europe, 1999–2002. Emerg Infect Dis 2004;10:1627–34.

[26] Wertheim HFL, Vos MC, Boelens HAM, et al. Low prevalence of methicillin-resistant *Staphylococcus aureus* (MRSA) at hospital admission in the Netherlands: the value of search and destroy and restrictive antibiotic use. J Hosp Infect 2004;56:321–5.

[27] Dailey L, Coombs GW, O'Brien FG, et al. Methicillin-resistant *Staphylococcus aureus*, western Australia. Emerg Infect Dis 2005;11:1584–90.

[28] Boyce JM, Potter-Bynoe G, Chenevert C, et al. Environmental contamination due to methicillin-resistant *Staphylococcus aureus*: possible infection control implications. Infect Control Hosp Epidemiol 1997;18:622–7.

[29] French GL, Otter JA, Shannon KP, et al. Tackling contamination of the hospital environment by methicillin-resistant *Staphylococcus aureus* (MRSA): a comparison between conventional terminal cleaning and hydrogen peroxide vapour decontamination. J Hosp Infect 2004;57:31–7.

[30] Wilson APR, Hayman S, Folan P, et al. Computer keyboards and the spread of MRSA. J Hosp Infect 2006;62:390–2.

[31] Garner JS. Guideline for isolation precautions in hospitals. Part I. Evolution of isolation practices, Hospital Infection Control Practices Advisory Committee. Am J Infect Control 1996;24:24–31.

[32] Pittet D. Hand hygiene: improved standards and practice for hospital care. Curr Opin Infect Dis 2003; 16:327–35.

[33] Boyce JM, Pittet D. Guideline for hand hygiene in health-care settings: recommendations of the Healthcare Infection Control Practices Advisory Committee and the HICPAC/SHEA/APIC/IDSA Hand Hygiene Task Force. Infect Control Hosp Epidemiol 2002;23(Suppl 12):S3–40.

[34] Gordin FM, Schultz ME, Huber RA, et al. Reduction in nosocomial transmission of drug-resistant bacteria after introduction of an alcohol-based handrub. Infect Control Hosp Epidemiol 2005;26: 650–3.

[35] Clancy M, Graepler A, Wilson M, et al. Active screening in high-risk units is an effective and cost-avoidant method to reduce the rate of methicillin-resistant *Staphylococcus aureus* infection in the hospital. Infect Control Hosp Epidemiol 2006;27: 1009–17.

[36] Jernigan JA, Clemence MA, Stott GA, et al. Control of methicillin-resistant *Staphylococcus aureus* at a university hospital: one decade later. Infect Control Hosp Epidemiol 1995;16:686–96.

[37] von Eiff C, Becker K, Machka K, et al. Nasal carriage as a source of *Staphylococcus aureus* bacteremia. N Engl J Med 2001;344(1):11–6.

[38] Shitrit P, Gottesman B, Katzir M, et al. Active surveillance for methicillin-resistant *Staphylococcus aureus* (MRSA) decreases the incidence of MRSA bacteremia. Infect Control Hosp Epidemiol 2006; 27:1004–8.

[39] Loveday HP, Pellowe CM, Jones SRLJ, et al. A systematic review of the evidence for interventions for the prevention and control of meticillin-resistant *Staphylococcus aureus* (1996–2004): report to the Joint MRSA Working Party (subgroup A). J Hosp Infect 2006;63(Suppl 1):S45–70.

[40] Cooper BS, Stone SP, Kibbler CC, et al. Isolation measures in the hospital management of methicillin resistant *Staphylococcus aureus* (MRSA): systematic review of the literature. BMJ 2004;329:533–8.

[41] Lines LA. Study of senior staff nurses' perceptions about MRSA. Nurs Times 2006;102:32–5.

[42] Johnson PDR, Martin R, Burrell LJ, et al. Efficacy of an alcohol/chlorhexidine hand hygiene program in a hospital with high rates of nosocomial methicillin-resistant *Staphylococcus aureus* (MRSA) infection. Med J Aust 2005;183(10):509–14.

[43] Rice LB. Antimicrobial resistance in gram-positive bacteria. Am J Med 2006;119(6 Suppl 1):S11–9.

[44] Fattom AI, Horwith G, Fuller S, et al. Development of StaphVAX, a polysaccharide conjugate vaccine against *S. aureus* infection: from the lab bench to phase III clinical trials. Vaccine 2004;22(7):880–7.

ELSEVIER
SAUNDERS

Crit Care Nurs Clin N Am 19 (2007) 69–75

CRITICAL CARE
NURSING CLINICS
OF NORTH AMERICA

Vancomycin-Resistant Enterococcus in Critical Care Areas

Sharon Bryant, MSN, ACNP[a,b,*], Jennifer Wilbeck, MSN, ACNP[a,c]

[a]Acute Care Nurse Practitioner Program, Vanderbilt University School of Nursing, 461 21st Avenue South, Nashville, TN 37240, USA
[b]Kindred Hospital, Nashville, TN, USA
[c]Centennial Medical Center Emergency Department, Nashville, TN, USA

Across the United States, infections resistant to conventional treatments are increasing at alarming rates. Vancomycin-resistant enterococci (VRE) are a particular emerging threat frequently encountered in critical care areas. Although the number of VRE infections continues to rise, available and effective treatments are not increasing at the same rate. Nurses working in these critical care areas are in a unique position to provide their patients with the care to prevent and treat VRE infections appropriately. To prevent and treat VRE infections, the critical care nurse must have an understanding of VRE, its origin, diagnosis, and management, and knowledge of strategies for surveillance and prevention.

Epidemiology

More than 2 million hospital-acquired infections are reported annually in the United States [1,2], with 12% occurring in ICUs [3]. Of the reported 2 million hospital-acquired infections, roughly 10% are related to VRE [4]. For patients in ICU settings, infection with VRE represents more than 25% of all nosocomial enterococcal infections [5] and is the third most common cause of bacteremia [6]. VRE bactermia increases length of stay in hospitals by an average of 2 weeks and carries an overall mortality rate of nearly 30% [7]. The financial costs of treatment for patients infected with VRE ranges from $17 to $29 billion dollars per year [1].

Enterococcus species are anaerobic gram-positive cocci that are found commonly as normal flora in the gastrointestinal tract. Enterococci have been shown to colonize on skin surfaces and in the genitourinary tract as well. Although there are are least 17 species of the genus Enterococcus, the most common enterococcal species related to infection and bacteremia are E faecium (85%–95%) and E faecalis (5%–10%) [7]. E faecium occurs more frequently as a nosocomial infection and carries a much higher mortality rate than infection with other enterococcal species [4]. Additionally, E faecium is the most common vancomycin-resistant Enterococcus species [8].

Numerous infections have been attributed to enterococci, including urinary tract infections, intra-abdominal abcesses, bacteremia, and endocarditis. Less commonly, meningitis and osteoarticular infections are attributed to enterococci [9]. Initially described in 1986, enterococci were the first organisms identified to show antibiotic resistance to vancomycin [10]. For patients who have community-acquired VRE, the most common sources are the gastrointestinal and genitourinary tracts. Common sources of nosocomial enterococcal bacteremia include central lines and intra-abdominal, surgical, and burn wounds as well as the gastrointestinal and genitourinary systems [4].

* Corresponding author. Vanderbilt University School Of Nursing, 461 21st Avenue South, Nashville, TN 37240.
  E-mail address: sharon.bryant@vanderbilt.edu (S. Bryant).

Risk factors

Risk factors for development of antimicrobial-resistant infections include severe illnesses, prolonged hospitalization, and overuse of broad-spectrum antibiotics [11,12]. Many argue that overprescribing of broad-spectrum antibiotics has led to increasing numbers of antimicrobial-resistant organisms. Researchers have shown that most patients who develop VRE bacteremias have undergone prior antibiotic therapy with cephalosporins, vancomycin, or agents with strong anaerobic coverage [9,13].

Antimicrobial resistance also has been attributed to the production of biofilm by microbial organisms. Biofilm is an aggregation of microbial cells to a surface located either inside or outside the body. The microbes form a semipermeable matrix composed mainly of polysaccharide material that allows microorganisms to immerse themselves in the polysaccharide medium and enhance their survival in unfavorable and stressful conditions. Biofilm production is a naturally occurring phenomenon that also contributes to decreased efficacy of antibiotics on particular bacteria, the emergence of antibiotic resistance, and the expression of antibiotic-resistant genes. The formation of biofilm by *E faecalis* has been derived from various isolates and has been shown to survive better in macrophages [14–16].

At the cellular level, the development of resistance by microbial organisms depends on the compatibility of the receptor sites between the antibiotic and the microorganism. The binding of vancomycin to a microorganism occurs between the D-alanine receptor sites of the two molecules. Under normal conditions, the D-alanine receptor site on the vancomycin molecule binds to the D-alanine receptor site on the microorganism. Chemical enzymatic reactions then catalyze the inhibition of cell wall synthesis and RNA production within the microbial cell. In vancomycin resistance, the D-alanine receptor site in the microbe is reconfigured to a D-lactate binding site. The vancomycin D-alanine receptor site and the D-lactate binding site on the microorganism are not compatible; therefore normal binding between the two molecules cannot occur. The end result is that vancomycin has no effect in inhibiting microbial replication and spread. The microbes are rendered resistant to the vancomycin molecule [17].

Numerous causes for the acquisition of VRE have been proposed and are listed in Box 1.

> **Box 1. Risk factors for the acquisition of vancomycin-resistant enterococci [7,11]**
>
> *General/environmental risk factors*
> High-volume use of broad-spectrum antimicrobial agents
> Patient overcrowding in facilities
> Understaffing of facilities
> Placement in ICU, transplant ward, or unit with high colonization pressure
>
> *Patient risk factors*
> Severity of illness
> Prolonged hospitalization
> Presence of indwelling catheters or invasive devices
> Prolonged mechanical ventilation
> Age
> Nonambulatory status
> Immunosuppression (including posttransplantation status)
> Diarrhea
> Renal insufficiency/chronic hemodialysis
> Proximity to patient who has VRE
>
> *Clinician risk factors*
> Poor adherence to infection-control practices
> Failure to recognize antimicrobial resistance in facility
> Use of contaminated equipment

Three specifically identified risk factors are considered: the patient's (1) environment, (2) level of immunocompromise, and (3) genetic predispositions. Colonization of VRE occurs more commonly among susceptible patients placed on units where colonization with VRE is higher, such as ICU or oncology units [8]. Patients who reside in a long-term care facility or nursing home or who are admitted to a hospital with more than 200 beds also have a higher risk of acquiring VRE [8,18]. The majority of patients in the ICU have central venous catheters that may serve as portals of entry for bacteria. Patients receiving total parenteral nutrition (TPN) have increased rates of VRE acquisition because the TPN mixture provides a medium for bacterial colonization and infection [19]. Patients in the ICU or those with a previous ICU admission are at a higher risk of VRE acquisition because they typically have higher rates of immunosuppression resulting from multiple comorbidities.

A key concept in understanding the risk for developing VRE centers on distinguishing VRE colonization from VRE infection. Colonization of VRE most commonly occurs within the gastrointestinal tract and almost always precedes infection. Colonization of the bacteria typically is asymptomatic and long-lived, with some studies documenting continued colonization for up to 1 year after the discontinuation of antibiotics [7]. The virulence of VRE allows the development of a reservoir for infectious spread either to other individuals or throughout the host's body in the setting of immunosuppression. Underlying infectious processes and immunosuppressive medications also have been shown to increase risk of VRE infection secondary to their immunosuppressive effects. In the ICU, patients infected with methicillin-resistant *Staphylococcus aureus* are at higher risk for VRE infections [20]. Patients who have weakened immune systems because of hematologic disorders, posttransplantation regimens, or severe illness are more likely to convert from a colonized state to infection with VRE [8].

The role that genetic predispositions play in VRE infections has a strong theoretical base. The *esp* gene has been identified in both human and animal specimens. Among the enterococcal species, only *E faecalis* has been found to carry the *esp* gene, which is thought to contribute to the emergence of antibiotic resistance. The *esp* gene is a large 1873–amino acid protein sequence expressed on the cell walls of bacteria. Expression of the *esp* gene enhances the production of biofilm by microorganisms and increases the affinity of biofilm attachment to polystyrene surfaces. Studies have shown that biofilm production is not limited to the enterococcal strains expressing the *esp* gene [14,16,21]. The issue of *esp* gene expression continues to be an area of scientific research and debate, and conflicting theories continue to be proposed.

Genes associated with specific vancomycin resistance include *vanA*, *vanB*, *vanC*, *vanD*, and *vanG*. These genes have been shown to reduce the affinity of vancomycin binding to the microbial receptor site. The specific mechanism of action and the origination of the *van* genes have yet to be determined, but the *van* gene is believed to have originated as a result of genetic transfer between humans.

Of the *van* genes, *VanB*, *vanD*, and *vanG* are highly prevalent in the human gastrointestinal tract and human rectal swabs. *VanA* has been linked to several *S aureus* isolates. *VanB* has been found mostly in anaerobic bacteria, whereas *VanD* and *VanG* have been identified in a few isolates of *E faecalis*. *VanC-1* has been identified specifically on *E gallinarum*. *VanC-2* and *VanC-3* have been identified specifically on *E casseliflavus*. The increased numbers of *van* genes carried on the surface of the microbes allow enhanced microbial resistance to vancomycin and the potential for multidrug resistance [22].

Diagnostics

Accurate and early detection of VRE colonization and infection is crucial to prevent the spread of the resistant microbe. Diagnosis typically is made by standard culture studies or by molecular techniques such as polymerase chain reaction (PCR) assays. PCR detects the presence of the *vanA* and *vanB* genes that are associated with VRE and is performed routinely on perianal, perirectal, and rectal swabs and stool specimens. Although positive results indicate colonization with VRE, these results alone are not diagnostic of infection. The use of PCR can reduce the time for detection of VRE from the 72 hours required for traditional cultures to less than 4 hours.

Although PCR testing is useful for rapid identification of VRE, there are circumstances in which it has been found to be unreliable. VRE may not be detected when the bacterial count in a specimen very low. Additionally, other organisms besides enterococci can express the *van* genes, leading to false-positive results. These two circumstances are rare, however, and PCR testing is used increasingly for detection of VRE [8].

Despite increased use of PCR testing, standard culture techniques are far from obsolete. Standard aerobic cultures, as well as broth or agar dilution tests, are used for antimicrobial susceptibility testing that would not be available with PCR techniques alone. Additionally, when investigating outbreaks of VRE, cultures allow detailed classification of enterococcal strains [7,8]. Both PCR testing and standard cultures are necessary components in the diagnosis of VRE.

Treatment

The goal for the initial treatment of VRE infection is to eradicate any sources of potential infection. For instance, abscesses should be drained, wounds must be débrided, and foreign bodies should be removed [7,9]. Numerous studies have demonstrated that bacteremia can be eradicated without the use of antimicrobial medications simply by removing an infected indwelling (eg, intravenous or urinary) catheter [9]. If these measures do not resolve the infection, treatment with antimicrobial agents may be indicated.

Antimicrobial medications must be reserved for patients who have VRE infection and who demonstrate active clinical evidence of infection, such as fever, chills, hypotension, and a positive blood culture from at least one peripheral blood draw [19]. As in treating all infections in critically ill patients, diligence is required to achieve maximized outcomes with minimal resistance. Limiting the use of extended-spectrum cephalosporins and antimicrobial agents with anaerobic coverage is critical in decreasing VRE colonization [9]. The Centers for Disease Control recently proposed guidelines for prevention and control of antimicrobial resistance [2]. The components of empiric antimicrobial treatment, ideal dosing, and duration of therapy have been well described by other authors [11,12,23]. Although few measures have substantial outcomes-based research studies to support their use, multiple treatment regimens have been proposed as effective against VRE infections.

One of the earliest drugs for treating VRE infections was quinupristin/dalfopristin, a bacteriostatic drug that became available in the United States in late 1999. Although the drug in vitro is effective in the treatment of *E faecium*, most *E faecalis* isolates and many other enterococci species are resistant to the drug [8,9]. The drug is available only parenterally, must be administered through a central line, and frequently causes myalgias and arthralgias. Use of quinupristin/dalfopristin has been called into question by multiple studies, two of which reported liver disease as a side effect [9,24]. Newer drugs including daptomycin and tigecycline show in vitro activity against VRE and have become available recently (in 2003 and 2005, respectively) but lack clinical data on success in treating VRE infections [8].

More extensively used in current critical care practice is linezolid, an oxazolidinone that became available in the United States in 2000. Linezolid binds to the 50s portion of the ribosomal subunit to prevent formation of the mRNA complex. Inhibition of the mRNA complex effectively inhibits DNA protein synthesis, making the drug bacteriostatic. Linezolid is available for both oral and parenteral routes with nearly equivalent bioavailabilities and is the only oral agent approved by the Food and Drug Administration for treatment of VRE infections. An additional benefit is that the drug has activity against *E faecium* as well as other enterococcal species (*E faecalis, E casseliflavus,* and *E gallinarum*). Numerous studies have documented linezolid's efficacy against multiple forms of enterococcal infections in varied clinical scenarios such as bacteremia, line sepsis, and endocarditis [9,25–27]. Thrombocytopenia tends to be the most commonly reported serious side effect. Unfortunately, emerging linezolid-resistant VRE infections have been reported [25,28,29].

Genitourinary infections with VRE are afforded additional therapeutic options that are ineffective for other systemic or solid-organ infections. Both fosomycin and nitrofurantoin achieve adequate therapeutic concentrations in urine but not in the blood and have been shown to be effective in small numbers of patients who have lower urinary tract VRE infections. Additionally, some fluoroquinolones have demonstrated in vitro activity against selected VRE isolates [9].

Debate continues regarding treatment for VRE colonization as a means to prevent VRE infection. Some researchers claim that treatment of colonized VRE may contribute to antibiotic resistance [20]. Theoretically, eliminating VRE colonization from susceptible hosts at high risk for infection may prove to be an effective prevention strategy. Potential patient populations that might benefit from decolonization include those with hematologic cancers and those who have received a stem cell transplant, patients in the ICU, liver transplant recipients, or patients receiving hemodialysis [9].

Several regimens for decolonization of the gastrointestinal tract have been described, including treatment with oral bacitracin, chloramphenicol, ramoplanin, doxycycline, gentamicin, tetracycline, rifampin, and novobiocin in multiple combinations [8,9,13]. Most promising for decolonization regimens seems to be ramoplanin, the first drug in the new glycolipodepsipeptide class of medications [9]. This bactericidal drug works by inhibiting cell wall synthesis and is effective against essentially all gram-positive bacteria. The drug is not absorbed systemically when taken orally and thus achieves high fecal drug concentrations with minimal side effects [9]. At this time, there is no effective antimicrobial agent available with strong support in the literature that can eradicate VRE colonization [8].

Prevention

With the limited number of effective therapeutic options, containing colonization and preventing the spread of VRE is crucial. Current research indicates that most enterococcal diseases probably spread from patient to patient through the hands of health care workers [7,20]. Prevention of VRE infections requires a multifaceted approach, including intensive infection control methodologies and aggressive surveillance strategies in addition to better antimicrobial prescribing practices. Due diligence in antimicrobial prescribing patterns also plays an essential role in preventing the development of VRE infections and all types of resistant organisms.

One method of infection control that has been identified for use in patients who have central venous catheters is the addition of positive-pressure mechanical valve (PPMV) ports. PPMV ports are needleless, closed system ports on the peripheral end of a catheter that may be accessed by a compatible blunt cannula injector or syringe alone. The ports typically are used for fluid and medication administration. When cleaned with an antimicrobial wipe such as alcohol before use, these closed systems are less likely to translocate bacteria from outside surfaces into the bloodstream, because only sterile fluids and medications are injected into the port. Several studies have demonstrated that the use of PPMV ports decreases the rate of central line infections and VRE bacteremia [30].

Strict contact isolation precautions have been described as essential in reducing transmission of VRE from colonized patients to susceptible hosts by the hands of health care workers [9,12]. As far back as the 1800s, hand washing was been identified as the most effective method of preventing the the transfer of organisms between persons. Modern health care workers, however, seem to fall short of even this most basic prevention strategy. Recent studies have demonstrated that only 20% to 48% of health care providers comply with hand washing protocols [1,31]. Based on mathematical formulations proposed in one study, a minimum compliance of 50% is required to control the spread of VRE throughout inpatient units [31]. Commonly cited reasons for lack of handwashing compliance are an increased workload for health care providers and the sense that there is little extra time to spend in this preventative intervention [1]. The recommended time required for effective hand washing is only 15 seconds.

Specific and exhaustive recommendations for effective hand washing that address technique as well as solutions used are described in the literature [32].

Other simple measures to prevent the spread of VRE include the use of isolation gowns, gloves, and face shields when performing patient care. Gloves should be changed if they tear or come into contact with body fluids, and all patient-care attire should be removed before leaving the room. Having equipment dedicated to the infected patient and assuring that all staff members comply with the isolation guidelines for that patient have been shown to decrease VRE transmission rates. Patients colonized or infected with VRE should be placed on contact isolation or in a semiprivate room with another patient also infected with VRE [9,20].

Debate exists regarding the expense associated with the use of isolation gowns for patients colonized with VRE. Many argue that the costs of the gown are prohibitive. In a 2004 study performed by Puzniak and colleagues [3], both infection and colonization rates were demonstrably lower when proper gowning techniques were used. The use of gowns to prevent VRE acquisition and infection resulted in a net hospital savings of about $420,000 related to the costs involved in the patient's length of stay and treatment for VRE infection [3]. Despite routine and correct use of contact precautions, a recent study by Duckro and colleagues [33] demonstrated spread of VRE from a contaminated to uncontaminated part of an ICU patient's room in nearly 1 out of every 10 patient encounters.

The use of active surveillance programs is another evidenced-based approach for preventing VRE transmission. Individual hospital units, entire health-care facilities, and even entire nations in which active surveillance programs are used have reported controlled nosocomial VRE infection rates [11]. One recent study reported that 86% of all VRE-colonized patients were identified only by the use of routine active surveillance cultures. These results suggest that cultures performed per standard protocol (ie, when patients seem to have a clinical infection) grossly underrepresent the number of patients colonized with VRE. Unidentified colonized patients continue to serve as a reservoir for spread of the resistant infection among patients [11]. A simple solution to this dilemma of patients who have unrecognized colonization seems to be the use of active surveillance programs.

There seems to be consensus within that literature that active surveillance efforts should be directed at least periodically toward high-risk patient populations. High-risk groups for colonization typically include patients in ICU, those in hematology and bone marrow suppression units, and those who have received a solid-organ transplant. Outpatient hemodialysis units also are included in routine surveillance attempts. Typically in these screenings stool rectal or perirectal cultures are obtained, and a routine schedule for their procurement seems to be standard [7]. Because less than half of VRE specimens are isolated from normally sterile body fluids such as blood and urine, some clinicians support routine culturing of all sterile and nonsterile clinical specimens (eg, catheter tips, sputum, stools, wound drainage) submitted to the laboratory [7].

Outcomes

Available studies report conflicting rates of morbidity and mortality for patients infected with VRE. Some researchers suggest that survival rates are lower and mortality rates are higher for patients who have VRE infections [10,24]. In 1998 Stosor and colleagues [34] reported that among patients with similar severity-of-illness scores, patients who had VRE bacteremia were more than four times more likely to die than those who had vancomycin-susceptible bacteremia. In a recent study that matched patient demographics, diagnoses, and illness severity, Song and colleagues [35] demonstrated that mortality rates were significantly higher in patients who had VRE bacteremia than in patients whose bacteremia was not caused by VRE. Another study reports that crude and infection-related mortality rates were higher among trauma patients who had VRE bacteremia than in matched control patients who had vancomycin-sensitive enterococcal infections [10].

Much recent research compares VRE infections with vancomycin-sensitive enterococcal infections [10]. These studies conclude that VRE is responsible for higher crude mortality rates, but the evidence to support VRE as an independent predictor of mortality has yet to be determined [10]. The documented higher mortality rates in VRE-infected patients and the recognized increased costs of caring for patients who have VRE necessitate the development of better surveillance techniques and additional effective therapeutic regimens.

Summary

Colonization with VRE must be identified to prevent the spread of the disease and the progression to infection in susceptible individuals. PCR assays and culturing techniques allow nurses and other members of the health care team to identify and treat colonized and infected patients. Although currently there is no effective treatment for VRE colonization, isolation precautions are paramount to prevent increased VRE transmission. Decolonization techniques should be considered in high-risk populations. For those who have clinical evidence of VRE infection, several approved treatment regimens can be implemented. The increasing incidence of VRE with simultaneous increasing resistance patterns demands the development of new antimicrobial agents. Collaborative management of both VRE colonization and infection can reduce the skyrocketing numbers of hospital acquired infections and mortality from VRE infections.

References

[1] Aragon D, Sole ML, Brown S. Outcomes of an infection prevention project focusing on hand hygiene and isolation practices. AACN Clin Issues 2005; 16(2):121–32.

[2] Diekema DJ, BootsMiller BJ, Vaughn TE, et al. Antimicrobial resistance trends and outbreak frequency in United States hospitals. CID 2004;38:78–85.

[3] Puzniak LA, Gillespie KN, Leet T, et al. A cost benefit analysis of gown use in controlling vancomycin resistant Enterococcus transmission: is it worth the price. Infect Control Hosp Epidemiol 2004;25(5): 418–24.

[4] de Piero M, Yarnold PR, Warren J, et al. Risk factors and outcomes associated with non-Enterococcus faecalis, non-Enterococcus faecium enterococcal bacteremia. Infect Control Hosp Epidemiol 2006; 27(1):28–33.

[5] Division of Healthcare Quality Promotion, National Center for Infectious Diseases, Centers for Disease Control and Prevention, Public Health Service, US Department of Health and Human Services. National Nosocomial Infections Surveillance (NNIS) Systems report: data summary from January 1992 through June 2003, issued August 2003. Am J Infect Control 2003;31:481–98.

[6] Raad II, Hend HA, Boktour M, et al. Vancomycin resistant Enterococcus faecium: catheter colonization, van gene and decreased susceptibility to antibiotics in biofilm. Antimicrob Agents Chemother 2005;49(12):5046–50.

[7] DeLisle S, Pel TM. Conundrums in the management of critically ill patients. Chest 2003;123(5):504S–18S.

[8] Zirakzadeh A, Patel R. Vancomycin-resistant enterococci: colonization, infection, detection and treatment. Mayo Clin Proc 2006;81(4):529–36.

[9] Kauffman CA. Therapeutic and preventative options for the management of vancomycin-resistant enterococcal infections. J Antimicrob Chemother 2003;51(Suppl S3):iii23–30.

[10] Lodise TP, McKinnin PS, Tam VH, et al. Clinical outcomes for patients with bacteremia caused by vancomycin resistant enterococcus in a level 1 trauma center. CID 2002;34:922–9.

[11] Salgado CD, O'Grady N, Farr BM, et al. Prevention and control of antimicrobial-resistant infections in intensive care patients. Crit Care Med 2005;33(10): 2373–82.

[12] Silveira F, Fujitani S, Paterson DL, et al. Antibiotic-resistant infections in the critically ill adult. Clin Lab Med 2004;24:329–41.

[13] Wong MT, Kauffman CA, Standiford HC, et al. Effective suppression of vancomycin-resistant enterococcus species in asymptomatic gastrointestinal carriers by a novel glycolipodepsipeptide, ramoplanin. CID 2001;33:1476–82.

[14] Raad II, Darouiche R, Haechem M, et al. Antibiotic colonization of catheters. Antimicrob Agents Chemother 1995;39:2397–400.

[15] Ramadhan AA, Hegedus E. Survivability of vancomycin resistant enterococci and fitness cost of vancomycin resistance acquisition. J Clin Pathol 2005; 58(7):744–6.

[16] Ramadhan AA, Hedegus E. Biofilm production and *esp* gene carriage in enterococci. J Clin Pathol 2005; 58(7):685–6.

[17] Levinson W, Jawetz E. Medical microbiology & immuniology. (CT): Appleton & Lange; 1998. p. 62–9.

[18] Polgreen PM, Beekman SE, Chen YY, et al. Epidemiology of methicillin resistant *Staphylococcus aureus* and vancomycin resistant *Enterococcus* in a rural state. Infect Control Hosp Epidemiol 2006; 27(3):252–6.

[19] Raad II, Hanna H, Boktour, et al. Catheter-related vancomycin resistant Enterococcus faecium bacteremia: clinical and molecular epidemiology. Infect Control Hosp Epidemiol 2005;26(7):658–61.

[20] Konegaard R, Myers F, Edward C. Arresting drug resistant organisms. Nursing 2005;35(6):48–50.

[21] Raad II, Hanna HA, Chaiban G, et al. The presence of the *esp* gene bioprosthetic colonization, and DNA restriction pattern in vancomycin-resistant *Enterococcus faecium* (VREF) causing catheter-related bacteremia (CRB). Presented at the 43rd Interscience Conference on Antimicrobial Agents and Chemotherapy. Chicago (IL), September 14–17, 2003.

[22] Domingo M-C, Huletsky A, Giroux R, et al. High prevalence of glycopeptide resistant genes vanB, vanD, and vanG not associated with enterococci in human fecal flora. Antimicrob Agents Chemother 2005;49(11):4784–6.

[23] Landman D, Quale JM. Management of infections due to resistant enterococci: a review of therapeutic options. J Antimicrob Chemother 1997;40: 161–70.

[24] Patel R. Clinical impact of vancomycin-resistant enterococci. J Antimicrob Chemother 2003; 51(Suppl S3):iii13–21.

[25] Birmingham MC, Rayner CR, Meagher AK, et al. Linezolid for the treatment of multidrug-resistant, gram-positive infections: experience from a compassionate-use program. CID 2003;36:159–68.

[26] Babcock HM, Ritchie DJ, Christiansen E, et al. Successful treatment of vancomycin-resistant enterococcus endocarditis with oral linezolid. CID 2001; 32:1373–5.

[27] Chien JW, Kucia ML, Salata RA, et al. Use of linezolid, an oxazolidinone, in the treatment of multidrug-resistant gram-positive bacterial infections. CID 2000;30:146–51.

[28] Gonzales RD, Schreckenberger PC, Graham FR, et al. Infections due to vancomycin-resistant Enterococcus faecium resistant to linezolid. Lancet 2001; 357:1179.

[29] Herrero IA, Issa NC, Patel R, et al. Nosocomial spread of linezolid-resistant, vancomycin resistant, vancomycin *Enterococcus faecium*. N Engl J Med 2002;346:867–9.

[30] Maragakis LL, Bradley KL, Song X, et al. Increased catheter related bloodstream infection rates after the introduction of a new mechanical valve intravenous access port. Infect Control Hosp Epidemiol 2006; 27(1):67–70.

[31] Austin DJ, Bonten JM, Weinstein RA, et al. Vancomycin-resistant enterococci in intensive-care hospital settings: transmission dynamics, persistence, and the impact of infection control programs. Proc Natl Acad Sci U S A 1999;96:6908–13.

[32] Vernon MO, Hayden MK, Trick WE, et al. Chlorhexidine gluconate to cleanse patients in a medical intensive care unit: the effectiveness of source control to reduce the bioburden of vancomycin resistant enterococci. Arch Intern Med 2006;166(3): 306–12.

[33] Duckro AN, Blom DW, Lyle EA, et al. Transfer of vancomycin resistant enterococci via health care worker hands. Arch Intern Med 2005;165(3): 302–7.

[34] Stosor V, Peterson LR, Postelnick M, et al. Enterococcus faecium bacteremia: does vancomycin resistance make a difference? Arch Intern Med 1998; 158:522–7.

[35] Song X, et al. Effect of nosocomial vancomycin resistant enterococcal bacteremia on mortality, length of stay and costs. Infect Control Hosp Epidemiol 2003;24:251–6.

ELSEVIER
SAUNDERS

CRITICAL CARE
NURSING CLINICS
OF NORTH AMERICA

Crit Care Nurs Clin N Am 19 (2007) 77–86

Sepsis in Critical Care

Joan E. King, PhD, RNC, ACNP, ANP

*Acute Care Nurse Practitioner Program, Vanderbilt University School of Nursing, 340 Frist Hall,
Nashville, TN 37240, USA*

Sepsis is a syndrome that reflects a constellation of signs and symptoms related to an infectious process that has accelerated in the inflammatory immune response, the coagulation and fibrinolytic pathways as well as endothelial changes. Conceptually sepsis is on a continuum that begins with the systemic inflammatory response syndrome (SIRS), and ends with multiple organ dysfunction syndrome (MODS) (Box 1).

The midpoints on the continuum are sepsis, severe sepsis, and septic shock. As Box 1 indicates, sepsis is clinically defined when a patient has met two of the stated criteria for SIRS and there is evidence of an infection or suspected infection [1]. Thus a patient may have a fever or be hypothermic, tachycardic, and/or tachypneic, have a partial pressure of carbon dioxide, arterial ($PaCO_2$) below 32 mm Hg, and/or have either an elevated white blood cell count (WBC) or a decreased WBC; or their bands could be 10%. Severe sepsis follows on the continuum with evidence of organ dysfunction that may include hypotension, oliguria, elevated lactate levels, or changes in mental status. Septic shock is defined clinically when the patient remains hypotensive despite fluid resuscitation [1]. In MODS multiple organs are dysfunctional despite fluid resuscitation, vasopressor therapy, and the use of positive inotropes.

Epidemiology of sepsis

The significance of sepsis becomes evident when the statistics are reviewed. It is estimated that 750,000 cases occur annually [2–4], with a mortality rate ranging from 30% to 50% [5–7]. Paz and Martin [3] indicate that sepsis is the

leading cause of death in "noncoronary" ICUs, and other researchers indicate it is the fourth leading cause of death in long-stay intensive care admissions [5]. Factors that have contributed to the rise in the incidence of sepsis include an increase in the elderly population who are at a higher risk because of underlying comorbidities and possibly incompetent inflammatory–immune systems, the increased incidence of resistant bacteria, and the increased use of invasive lines that provide a portal of entry for bacteria and other pathogens.

Previously sepsis was associated with gram-negative infections, but current data indicate that between one third and one half of all cases of sepsis are the related to gram-positive infections [5]. Together gram-negative and gram-positive infections account for approximately 85% of all cases [5]. Five percent of the cases are attributed to fungal infections, including Candida, which has a 40% mortality rate [8].

Just as there is a critical window of opportunity for treatment for myocardial infarctions or strokes, sepsis has a 6-hour window of opportunity for stabilization that impacts the mortality and morbidity data [9]. Within the 6-hour treatment window, the first hour is the pivotal period for early treatment [5,10,11]. Because of the data supporting the importance of early recognition and initiation of treatment, patients who are at risk for developing sepsis should be monitored closely. This population includes patients who have other comorbidities such as type 1 or type 2 diabetes, patients who have chronic renal failure, and individuals who are immunosuppressed (including patients who have cancer or HIV, individuals receiving steroid therapy, posttransplantation patients, the elderly, and the very young). Trauma patients (including burn patients), patients undergoing abdominal surgery, postpartum patients,

E-mail address: joan.king@vanderbilt.edu

doi:10.1016/j.ccell.2006.10.007

Box 1. Definition of terms [1,2]

Systemic inflammatory response syndrome (SIRS) manifested by two or more of the following clinical signs:
Temperature >38°C or <36°C
Heart rate >90 beats/min
Respiratory rate >20 breaths/min or arterial partial pressure of carbon dioxide ($Paco_2$) <32 mm Hg
White blood cell count >12,000/mm^3 or < 4000/mm^3 or > 10% immature (band) forms

Sepsis: SIRS with evidence or suspected evidence of infection and at least two of the following:
Temperature >38°C or <36°C
Heart rate >90 beats/minute
Respiratory rate >20 breaths/min or $Paco_2$ <32 mm Hg
White blood cell count >12,000/mm^3 or <4000/mm^3 or >10% immature (band) forms

Severe sepsis: sepsis with evidence of end-organ dysfunction
Hypotension or hypoperfusion
Lactic acidosis
Oliguria
Acute changes in mental status

Septic shock: severe sepsis that is refractory to fluid resuscitation

Multiple organ dysfunction syndrome (MODS): dysfunction of multiple organs requiring fluid, vasopressor, and positive inotropic support.

Box 2. Diagnoses placing patients at increase risk for developing sepsis

Diabetes mellitus (type 1 or type 2)
Chronic renal failure
Immunosuppressive therapy
  Cancer
  Steroid therapy
  HIV
  Posttransplantation
Extremes of age (elderly or the very young)
Trauma
Burns
Abdominal surgery
Postpartum status
Meningitis

and glucose to the cells and the availability of neutrophils, macrophages, and other mediators to the area of injury to contain and eradicate any bacteria or foreign body. An increase in vascular permeability also facilitates the delivery of oxygen, glucose, neutrophils, and macrophages to the needed area. Cellular activation is the activation of neutrophils and macrophages to phagocytose any foreign substances or debris and to begin the process of microdébridement of the involved area. Activation of the clotting cascade facilitates the walling off of the injured area and minimizes any blood loss. The IIR is meant to protect the host, limit the extent of the injury, and promote wound healing. It is meant to be a controlled response in proportion to the body's needs.

Pathophysiology of sepsis

In sepsis, the normal IIR is accelerated or increased, and the normal anti-inflammatory functions cease to operate. The chemical mediators or cytokines, which typically are a protective mechanism that facilitates the destruction of bacteria or any foreign substance by vasodilation, increased vascular permeability, activation of neutrophils and macrophages, and activation of the coagulation cascade, begin to function out of control. Rather than an organized process that is reduced by the activation of anti-inflammatory agents once the infection has been resolved, in sepsis the process proceeds unchecked [12]. Initially, as the process starts, a patient may exhibit signs of SIRS. The patient may present initially

and individuals who have meningitis also are at risk of becoming septic (Box 2) [1]. Once the septic process begins, 20% of the individuals progress to severe sepsis, and 46% develop septic shock [12].

Physiology of the inflammatory immune response

To understand sepsis, it is important to understand the body's normal response to infection, which is the inflammatory immune response (IIR). The IIR, which normally is controlled by the complement system, involves four major components: vasodilation, increased vascular permeability, cellular activation, and coagulation. Vasodilation increases the availability of oxygen with tachycardia and tachypnea, and the WBC may be either elevated or depressed (see Box 1). At this point the IIR has become overly activated, but a source of infection has yet to be identified. As the infection becomes evident, the heart rate may increase, and the respiratory rate remains greater than 20 breaths per minute, with a resulting decrease in the $Paco_2$ as the minute ventilation increases and carbon dioxide is "blown off." The WBC again may be elevated ($> 12,000$ mm^3) or decreased (< 4000 mm^3), and a source of infection is either confirmed or strongly suspected.

Pathophysiologically, the chemical mediators produced by the complement system and the IIR begin to escalate the normal inflammatory response. Specific chemical mediators that are linked to the development of sepsis include cytokines such as tumor necrosis factor alpha, platelet-activating factor, interleukin-1, interleukin-6, interleukin-12, arachidonic acid metabolites (including leukotrienes, prostaglandins, and thromboxane A_2), oxygen radicals, nitric oxide, and proteases [2,5,6]. Activation of these mediators stimulates neutrophils, macrophages, monocytes, endothelial cells, and platelets. These cells in turn stimulate the continued release of the added chemical mediators that then stimulate more neutrophils, macrophages, and monocytes and also the clotting cascade with the stimulation of platelets and clot formation, the fibrinolytic system, and endothelial cell changes (Table 1). As the clotting cascade accelerates in activity, it contributes to the stimulation of more inflammatory cells including T and B cells, causing the release of more chemical mediators, and a self-perpetuating cycle develops. Activation of the inflammatory cells produces the release of more chemical mediators; more chemical mediators stimulate the clotting cascade; and the clotting cascade stimulates both the fibrinolytic process and continued activation of the inflammatory cells. The self-perpetuating process continues unchecked and out of control.

Other unique aspects of the septic process include an increased expression of neutrophils [13], and their lifespan is prolonged beyond the typical 6- to 10-hour period. This phenomenon contributes to both the acceleration of the IIR and the magnitude of the response: more neutrophils are recruited during the septic process, and they are more active for a longer period of time.

Table 1
Components contributing to the self-perpetuating cycle of sepsis

Complement system	Target	Outcome
Enzyme cascade of 20+ proteins	Inflammatory immune system	Vasodilation
		Increased capillary permeability
		Increased phagocytic activity of leukocytes
		Increased release of toxic by- products
		Cardiovascular instability
		Endothelial damage
		Clotting abnormalities
		Tissue and organ damage of the lungs, vasculature, kidneys, and liver
Leukocytes Neutrophils Macrophages Monocytes	Increased phagocytic activity produces excessive release of proteases, oxygen free radicals, tumor necrosis factor, platelet-activating factor, interleukin-1, arachidonic acid metabolites	Increased capillary permeability Interstitial edema Activation of the clotting cascade Microthrombi Vasodilation Organ dysfunction
Platelets	Inflammatory immune system Clotting cascade	Increased platelet aggregation Neutrophil activation Increased capillary permeability Microthrombi Vasoconstriction
Endothelial cells	Damage to endothelial cells	Increased capillary permeability Acceleration of the clotting cascade

In sepsis the responses no are longer localized to a specific region or area of injury; rather, it is a systemic process. The patient systemically vasodilates and becomes hypotensive. Also, the systemic vascular resistance decreases [14]. As the systemic vascular resistance decreases, the patient becomes more refractory to normal fluid replacement. The increase in vascular permeability also is a systemic process, and it is enhanced by chemically mediated endothelial cell damage. The systemic increase in vascular permeability accounts for the fluid shifts from the intravascular space into the interstitial spaces. The result is generalized edema [12]. Acceleration of the clotting cascade results in the formation of fibrin threads that begin to occlude the microvasculature [12]. The increase in fibrin production then accelerates fibrinolysis, placing the patient at increased risk for both clot formation and bleeding [12]. The combination of the drop in the systemic vascular resistance, the fluid shifts into the interstitial spaces, and the deposition of fibrin in the microvasculature leads to hypoperfusion of the body's organs. Hypoperfusion of the organs then leads to organ dysfunction and ultimately to organ failure. It is important to recognize that, because sepsis is a systemic process, all organs are affected in varying degrees, and it is paramount for the nurse to monitor the septic patient closely for the development of MODS (Box 3) [4,6,15].

Assessment

Although monitoring for MODS is critical for the septic patient, identifying patients at risk for sepsis is equally important (see Box 2). Targeting patients at risk and performing ongoing assessments to identify early physiologic changes is

a critical step in the management of septic patients (Box 4) [1]. These changes include subtle alterations in level of conscious, the development of a fever, and an increase in the respiratory rate [4,5,15]. An elevated lactate level or hyperlactatemia (>2 mEq/L), which may occur because of the liver's inability to clear the blood or because of the maldistribution of blood, also may signal sepsis [9,11,14]. Other markers that may signal sepsis are elevations in C-reactive protein and procalcitonin [10]. Both are biologic markers, but procalcitonin rises faster than C-reactive protein and clears more quickly once an inflammatory process subsides. Procalcitonin has 100% sensitivity but only 72% specificity [10], making it an acceptable marker for the inflammatory process but not a diagnostic marker for sepsis.

Common sources of infection triggering the sepsis syndrome include the lungs, abdominal wounds, and urinary tract infections [12]. Consequently during the early resuscitation phase, sputum, wound, and urine cultures are essential. Although only 30% to 50% of the patients who have severe sepsis or are in septic shock have a positive blood culture [10], blood cultures are critical for determining appropriate antibiotic therapy. It is recommended that two cultures be drawn simultaneously from two different venipuncture sites or from a central venous access device and a peripheral site if the central venous access line is more than 48 hours old [9,10]. The International Sepsis Forum Consensus Conference recommends that at least 10 mL of blood be obtained for each sample [16]. If a patient has more than one central venous access site, a culture should be obtained from each site. Obtaining multiple cultures from different sites simultaneously helps the clinician confirm the causative agent and also the source of the infection. Positive blood cultures for the same organism obtained from different sites help confirm the causative agent. If the central venous access culture is positive and the percutaneous sample is negative, the central access device should be considered as the source of the infection, and replacement is needed. In addition to blood cultures, a sputum culture, a urine culture, and any wound or drainage cultures should be obtained before antibiotic therapy is begun. If the patient is stable enough for transport, a CT scan may be helpful in identifying any internal pockets of infection. If the patient is too unstable for transport, Dellinger and colleagues [9] recommend an ultrasound study to rule out any other sources of infection.

Box 3. Complications related to sepsis and septic shock: end-organ dysfunction

Acute lung injury
Acute respiratory distress syndrome
Low cardiac output syndrome
Acute renal failure
Liver failure
Disseminated intravascular coagulation
Stroke
Ischemic bowel

Box 4. Assessment parameters

Neurologic assessment
Level of consciousness
Orientation
Pupillary check
Glasgow Coma Scale

Cardiovascular assessment
Heart rate and rhythm
Presence of ectopy
Central venous pressure
Jugular venous distension)
  Systolic and diastolic arterial
    pressure
  Mean arterial pressure
  Hemodynamic monitoring
    Cardiac output
    Cardiac index
    Pulmonary artery occlusive
      pressure
    Systemic vascular resistance
    Mixed venous oxygen saturation
  Presence and quality of peripheral
    pulses
  Capillary refill
  Skin color and temperature (mottling
    and coolness of extremities)

Respiratory assessment
Respiratory rate
Quality of breath sounds (anterior and
  posterior)
Arterial oxygen saturation
Arterial blood gases
Use of accessory muscles
Ventilator settings:
  Mode of ventilation
  Rate (spontaneous and ventilator
    rate)
  Positive end-expiratory pressure
  Tidal volume
  Peak inspiratory pressure
Shunting: Pao_2/Fio_2 (<300 indicates acute
  lung injury; <200 indicates acute
  respiratory distress syndrome)

Gastrointestinal and hepatic assessment
Presence or absence of bowel sounds
Percussion: tympany versus dullness
Abdomen: soft, firm, or distended
Hepatomegaly
Liver enzymes: alanine aminotransferase
  and aspartate aminotransferase

Bilirubin
Presence of nausea, vomiting, or
  diarrhea
Gastric residuals if receiving tube
  feedings

Renal assessment
Urinary output hourly and every 8 hours
Color, smell, and presence of sediment
  in the urine
Serum urea nitrogen, creatinine
Creatinine clearance: should be
  evaluated before antibiotics are
  administered

Hematologic assessment
Hematocrit/hemoglobin
White blood cell count with differential
Prothrombin time with international
  normalized ration
Partial thromboplastin time
Platelets
If disseminated intravascular coagulation
  is suspected, assess for
    Central catheter insertion sites: oozing
    Presence of petechiae
    D-dimer test

*Integument assessment and sources
of infection*
Indwelling catheters or central venous
  access devices
Wounds and drainage for evidence
  of infection, purulent drainage
Decubitus ulcers
Sinusitis
Cellulitis
Urinary tract infection

Endocrine
Glucose levels
Adrenal function if adrenal insufficiency
  is suspected

Pain and anxiety (if providing sedation)
Richmond Agitation Sedation Scale
Restlessness
Complaints of pain or anxiety

Treatment

Specific treatment recommendations have emerged from the Surviving Sepsis Campaign II conference, which was an international effort including 11 different organizations and focusing on evidence-based practices for the management of sepsis [9]. The Surviving Sepsis Campaign II conference concluded that early treatment is pivotal to improve outcomes related to sepsis and septic shock [9,11]. Treatment should begin even as the patient presents in the emergency department [17]. The goal within the first 6 hours of presentation is to achieve a central venous pressure (CVP) of 8 to 12 mm Hg, a mean arterial pressure (MAP) of 65 mm Hg or greater, a urinary output (UOP) of 0.5 mL/kg/h or greater, and a central venous (superior vena cava) or mixed venous oxygen saturation of 70% or greater (Box 5) [9]. Initial therapy to achieve these goals is fluid resuscitation, with rates of 40 to 60 mL/kg/h as appropriate volume replacement [9]. If the targets for the MAP and UOP are not met, it is recommended that the patient receive packed red blood cells to achieve a hematocrit of 30% or more or that a dobutamine infusion be initiated if low cardiac output is suspected [9].

The Surviving Sepsis Campaign II conference recommended that antibiotics be started within 1 hour of recognition of the syndrome [8,9]. For emergency departments and some critical care units, having premixed antibiotics available may facilitate timely administration. Factors that must be considered when selecting antibiotic coverage include the patient's probable diagnosis or source of infection, the patient's prehospital environment, the prevalence and susceptibility pattern of the hospital, and any drug intolerances or allergies the patient may have. A broad-spectrum antibiotic or antibiotics that address these criteria should be administrated. Evidence-based data indicate that monotherapy with a third- or fourth-generation cephalosporin may be used, or combination therapy using one beta-lactam antibiotic and an aminoglycoside may be given [5,8,9]. Once culture results are available, antibiotic coverage should be targeted to the specific organisms identified. Appropriate antibiotic

coverage with the proper drug and dosage has been shown to reduce mortality from 34% to 18% [5,8]. Antibiotic coverage should begin with a loading dose, but dosages must be adjusted appropriately if the patient demonstrates any hepatic or renal dysfunction [9]. If vancomycin, gentamicin, or tobramycin is selected for treatment, trough levels must be monitored because nephrotoxicity is positively correlated with prolonged elevated trough levels [10].

In addition to obtaining cultures, and based on diagnostic studies such as a CT or ultrasound scan, identified areas of infection should be débrided or drained. The Surviving Sepsis Campaign II conference calls this procedure "source control" [9,18]. Because the underlining derangement in sepsis is an accelerated self-perpetuating inflammatory response, removing the source of the problem is pivotal. In some instances source control may require surgical resection of ischemic bowel, the drainage of abscesses, or the removal of infected access devices.

To date there is no strong research supporting the use either colloid or crystalloid fluids [9,14]. The European community supports the use of colloids, whereas providers in the United States gravitate toward crystalloids [14]. Economics does play a role in these decisions. Crystalloids are far less expensive than colloids, but typically three times the volume of crystalloids, in comparison to colloids, is required to achieve the same target goals. Crystalloids also produce more edema, caused by the translocation of fluids into the interstitial spaces [9,14]. Regardless of the fluid selected, initial administration of fluids should consist of a 30-minute bolus of either 500 to 1000 mL of a crystalloid or 300 to 500 mL of a colloid [9,14]. Monitoring CVP, UOP, and MAP provides the guidelines to determine whether the initial resuscitation has been successful [9,19]. Because many septic patients have other comorbidities, assessing fluid overload is important also. Cardiac output may decrease if the patient has congestive heart failure and the preload exceeds their therapeutic range. Because fluid has backed up into the pulmonary bed, the MAP does not rise, the CVP is elevated, and the patient begins to develop signs and symptoms of pulmonary congestion and pulmonary edema.

As previously stated, if the target goals listed in Box 5 are not met with adequate fluid resuscitation, vasopressor therapy should be instituted. The Surviving Sepsis Campaign II conference recommended either norepinephrine or dopamine for

---

Box 5. Target goals for treatment within the first six hours

Central venous pressure of 8–12 mm Hg
Mean arterial pressure ≥65 mm Hg
Urinary output ≥0.5 mL/kg/h
Central venous (superior vena cava)
   or mixed venous oxygen saturation
   ≥70%

vasopressor therapy. The use of low-dose dopamine is not recommended, however. Studies comparing low-dose dopamine with placebo indicated no difference in outcome [9]. If the patient has a low cardiac output and remains hypotensive, dobutamine may be added to the regimen as a positive inotrope [9].

The use of steroids has been an ongoing controversy since the 1980s. Current recommendations are to use hydrocortisone, 200 to 300 mg/d in divided doses or continuous infusion for 7 days, for patients who have septic shock and who are refractory to both fluid resuscitation and vasopressor support [9]. If adrenal insufficiency has been identified, steroid replacement is appropriate also [20]. High-dose steroid therapy is contraindicated, however. Studies have shown it to be ineffective and in some cases detrimental [9]. For individuals who are septic but are not in septic shock, steroids are not recommended unless the patient has a comorbidity that merits their use.

One of the newest medications supported by clinical trials (including the Recombinant Human Activated Protein C Worldwide Evaluation in Severe Sepsis study) is recombinant human activated protein C (rhAPC) [15,21,22]. Because of the acceleration of the clotting cascade and the decreased rate of fibrinolysis, patients in severe sepsis or septic shock produce fibrin threads that occlude the microvasculature, contributing to further organ dysfunction and failure. rhAPC is an anticoagulant that also has anti-inflammatory and profibrinolytic properties. Studies have demonstrated its efficacy in patients who have severe sepsis, sepsis-induced acute respiratory distress syndrome, or septic shock with an Acute Physiology and Chronic Health Evaluation II score of 25 or higher [21,22]. Because rhAPC is an anticoagulant, it is contraindicated in patients who are at risk for bleeding. Individuals in whom it should not be used include those who are actively bleeding, who have had a hemorrhagic stroke in the past 3 months, who have experienced severe head trauma or intracranial or intraspinal surgery within the past 2 months or other trauma involving the risk of severe bleeding, who have an epidural catheter, or who have an intracranial mass or lesion or evidence of herniation [9].

The use of blood and blood products is another area that has undergone significant changes. Research from the Transfusion Requirements in Critical Care Trial indicates that a hemoglobin between 7 and 9 g/dL is adequate for critically ill patients [9,15]. Based on these data,

the recommendation of the Surviving Sepsis Campaign II conference is to transfuse a septic patient only when the hemoglobin is below 7 g/dL [9,23]. The exception to this recommendation is to transfuse a patient with packed red blood cells to a hematocrit of 30% if the central venous saturations have remained low during initial resuscitation [9]. The recommendation is to administer fresh frozen plasma products only when there is evidence of active bleeding or when bleeding is anticipated during surgery and the laboratory data document an increased prothrombin time, international normalized ratio, or partial thromboplastin time. If a patient's platelets are below 5000/mm^3, platelets should be administered even if the patient presents with no evidence of bleeding. Platelet levels between 5000/mm^3 and 30,000/mm^3 may require replacement if the patient is at risk for bleeding [9,23]. Patients with platelet levels greater than 50,000/mm^3 should receive additional platelets only if they are actively bleeding or are scheduled for a surgical procedure.

Whether they developed acute respiratory distress syndrome or acute lung injury before becoming septic, or because their lung injury is the result of sepsis, many patients require mechanical ventilation. Evidence-based practice recommends the use of low tidal volumes (6 mL/kg) and low levels of positive end-expiratory pressures while maintaining end-inspiratory plateau pressures less than 30 cm H_2O [9]. The use of low tidal volumes may lead to an elevated $PaCO_2$ level or what is termed "permissive hypercapnia." Except for patients who have increased intracranial pressures, allowing the $PaCO_2$ to rise above normal values seems less harmful than the barotrauma that can develop from large tidal volumes [24,25].

If a patient requires intubation and mechanical ventilation, semirecumbent positioning is recommended to reduce the incidence of aspiration and subsequent ventilator-acquired pneumonia. It also is recommended that ventilated patients undergo a daily spontaneous breathing trial once they are hemodynamically stable without vasopressors, their arterial oxygen saturation values are stable on low levels of positive end-expiratory pressures, and they no longer require high levels of oxygen [9]. Because intubation and mechanical ventilation can be perceived as a stress, research supports the use of sedation and analgesia. Neuromuscular blockades are not recommended, however. The Surviving Sepsis Campaign II conference recommended the implementation of a sedation protocol that sets specific sedation goals and allows intermittent lightening or interruption of an infusion to reassess the patient [9,26]. Many sedation scales are available. The Richmond Agitation Sedation Scale is one standardized tool that allows the nurse to titrate a patient's sedation to a desired level of sedation [26].

Another new focus in the management of septic patients is glycemic control. Based on the research started by Van den Berge [27], maintaining serum blood glucose levels within normal limits reduces mortality and morbidity for intensive care patients. Although Van den Berge's work focused on maintaining glucose levels between 80 and 110 mg/dL, the Surviving Sepsis Campaign II conference's present recommendation is to maintain a glucose level below 150 mg/dL in an effort to avert episodes of hypoglycemia [1,9]. Because the stress response promotes hyperglycemia, achieving glycemic control requires the use of a continuous insulin infusion, and hourly or every-30-minute glucose monitoring to titrate the infusion rate and prevent possible hypoglycemia [28].

Although septic patients present many unique aspects to the care because of the overstimulation of their inflammatory response, the clotting cascade and fibrinolytic process, and changes in their endothelial cells, these patients also require the same fundamental treatment that other critically ill patients require. These measures include maintaining adequate nutrition (using the gut if it is functional) and prophylaxis for deep vein thrombosis (DVT). Because septic patients frequently have more than one risk factor for the development of a DVT, the use of either low-dose unfractionated heparin or low-molecular-weight heparin (enoxaparin) is recommended [9,29]. If unfractionated heparin is selected, administration of heparin three times a day is recommended; enoxaparin can be administered once a day [29]. If a patient is at high risk for bleeding, and heparin or enoxaparin cannot be used, compression stockings and/or an intermittent compression device are recommended [9,29]. In addition, because of the increased production of gastric secretions associated with the stress response, all septic patients should receive stress ulcer prophylaxis. Presently the recommendation is to use H_2 receptor blockers, because no evidenced-based research supports the use of proton-pump inhibitors versus H_2 receptor blockers [9,29].

Caring for a patient who has sepsis or septic shock requires continual vigilance for what is termed "end organ damage" (see Box 3). As previously stated, the septic process is systemic, not isolated to any particular organ. Because the chemical mediators or cytokines circulate and continue to activate neutrophils, macrophages, platelets, and the clotting cascade and produce additional endothelial damage, organ dysfunction and failure ensue. The heart, lungs, kidneys, liver, brain, hematologic system, and gut are all susceptible to organ failure. A number of the chemical mediators, including platelet-activating factor, interleukin-1, and leukotrienes, directly produce myocardial depression [2]. The nurse at the bedside and other practitioners must assess the patient continually for signs and symptoms of heart failure or low cardiac output syndrome, acute lung injury or acute respiratory distress syndrome, hepatic failure, acute renal failure, ischemic bowel, coagulopathies, and strokes secondary to hemorrhage or emboli (see Box 4) [4,19]. Cardiovascular stability needs to be monitored hourly including hemodynamic assessments along with assessment of oxygen delivery and oxygen consumption through the monitoring for arterial oxygen saturation and mixed venous oxygen saturation. It is critical to monitor laboratory data indicating liver function (aspartate aminotransferase and alanine aminotransferase) as well as chemistry panels that monitor potassium, sodium chloride, serum urea nitrogen, and creatinine and coagulation indices (prothrombin time, partial thromboplastin time, platelets, hematocrit, and hemoglobin). Because of the involvement of the clotting cascade and the reduced activity of the fibrinolysis system, 20% of septic patients develop disseminated intravascular coagulation (DIC) [4]. Many times the initial sign of DIC is bleeding or oozing from puncture sites, including vascular access sites. The development of DIC can be confirmed by monitoring of D-dimer levels. D-dimers are a cross-linked fibrin degradation product and indicate the plasmin lysis of a fibrin clot. A positive D-dimer test has a high sensitivity for DIC, although not a high specificity. The test also may be positive secondary to a pulmonary embolus or DVT or other clot formation. Clinical signs and symptoms of bleeding combined with a positive D-dimer test confirm the diagnosis of DIC [30]. The development of DIC signals additional microvasculature impairment secondary to microthrombi. As the microthrombi occlude blood flow both to and within organs, further organ damage and failure ensues. Frequently the end result is MODS, in which individual organs no longer can function adequately, and failure and death ensue. Because of the high mortality rate associated with DIC and MODS, research efforts in sepsis have focused on preventing the escalating picture of failure. Therefore, the goal is to achieve stabilization within the first 6 hours after the diagnosis of septic syndrome.

Threaded throughout the entire care of septic patients is the fundamental need to address their psychosocial concerns. Frequently these patients present to the emergency department or have been hospitalized for other reasons, and their clinical course has deteriorated rapidly. As their condition deteriorates, evidence-based protocols focus on the need for timely assessment of their condition, the need for multiple cultures and rapid fluid resuscitation, and the need to begin antibiotic therapy quickly. Often the patient is intubated and mechanically ventilated quickly. For both the patient and the family, this process becomes a crisis that can escalate if the patient's and the family's psychosocial needs are not addressed [4]. The patient and the family must be informed of the changes in care and the rationale behind the changes, and end-of-life issues must be addressed also. The goal of health care providers is to provide the best care possible and to help the patient achieve an optimal outcome. The patient's goals must be assessed and addressed appropriately, including their wishes related to mechanical ventilation and cardiopulmonary resuscitation. With advances in treatment and in prevention of complications, the survival rates for sepsis and septic shock will improve, but it is vital that nurses include both the patient and the family in the decision-making process.

Summary

Sepsis is a syndrome produced by the accelerated activity of the inflammatory immune response, the clotting cascade, and endothelial damage. It is a systemic process that can progress easily into septic shock and MODS. The chemical mediators or cytokines produce a complex self-perpetuating process that impacts all body systems. It is critical for the nurse first to identify patients at risk for developing sepsis and to assess patients who have SIRS and sepsis continually for signs and symptoms of organ involvement and organ dysfunction. Once sepsis has been diagnosed, evidence-based practice indicates initiation of fluid resuscitation. Vasopressor therapy, positive inotropic support, and appropriate antibiotic therapy should be started within the first hour. Within a 6-hour timeframe the goal is stabilization of the CVP, MAP, and UOP to prevent further organ damage. The challenge for nurses caring for septic patients is to support the treatment goals, to prevent added complications including stress ulcers, DVTs, aspiration pneumonia, and the progression to MODS, and to address the patient's and the family's psychosocial needs. As complex as the pathophysiology of sepsis is, the nursing care is equally complex but also rewarding. Patients who previously might have died now recover as vigilant nursing care combines forces with new drug therapies and evidence-based practice guidelines.

References

[1] O'Hanlon K, Ferri F, Kim A, et al. Sepsis. Available at: www.firstconsult.com. Accessed July 16, 2006.

[2] Sommers M. The cellular basis of septic shock. Crit Care Nurs Clin North Am 2003;15(1):13–25.

[3] Paz H, Martin A. Sepsis in an aging population. Crit Care Med 2006;34(1):234–5.

[4] Kleinpell R. The role of the critical care nurse in the assessment and management of the patient with severe sepsis. Crit Care Nurs Clin North Am 2003; 15(1):27–34.

[5] Hanna N. Sepsis and septic shock. Top Emerg Med 2003;25(2):158–65.

[6] Gilroy D, Vallance P. Resolution of sepsis. Circulation 2005;111(1):2–4.

[7] Marshall J, Vincent J, Guyatt G, et al. Outcome measures for clinical research in sepsis: a report of the 2nd Cambridge Colloquium of the International Sepsis Forum. Crit Care Med 2005;33(8):1708–16.

[8] Bochud P, Bonten M, Marchetti O, et al. Antimicrobial therapy for patients with severe sepsis and septic shock: an evidence-based review. Crit Care Med 2004;32(11):S495–512.

[9] Dellinger RP, Carlet J, Masur H, et al. Surviving sepsis campaign guidelines for management of severe sepsis and septic shock. Crit Care Med 2004; 32(3):858–73.

[10] Cohen J, Brun-Buisson C, Torres A, et al. Diagnosis of infection in sepsis: an evidence-based review. Crit Care Med 2004;32(11):S466–94.

[11] Rhodes A, Bennett E. Early goal-directed therapy: an evidence- based review. Crit Care Med 2004; 32(11):S448–50.

[12] Braun L, Cooper L, Malatestinic W, et al. A sepsis review: epidemiology, economics and disease characteristics. Dimens Crit Care Nurs 2003;22(3): 117–24.

[13] Marshall J. Neutrophils in the pathogenesis of sepsis. Crit Care Med 2005;33(12):S502–5.

[14] Vincent J, Gerlach H. Fluid resuscitation in severe sepsis and septic shock: an evidence-based review. Crit Care Med 2004;32(11):S451–4.

[15] Kleinpell R. Working out the complexities of severe sepsis. Nurs Pract 2005;30(4):43–8.

[16] Calandra T, Cohen J. The International Sepsis Forum Consensus Conference on Definitions of Infection in the Intensive Care Unit. Crit Care Med 2005;33(7):1538–48.

[17] Maynard A. Surviving sepsis: standard protocols improve outcomes. J Emerg Nurs 2006;32(1):9–10.

[18] Marshall JC, Maier RV, Jimenez M, et al. Source of control in the management of severe sepsis and septic shock: an evidence-based review. Crit Care Med 2004;32(11):S513–26.

[19] Levy M, Macias W, Vincent J, et al. Early changes in organ function predict eventual survival in severe sepsis. Crit Care Med 2005;33(10):2194–201.

[20] Keh D, Sprung CL. Use of corticosteroid therapy in patients with sepsis and septic shock: an evidence-based review. Crit Care Med 2004;32(11):S527–33.

[21] Angus D, Laterre P, Helterbrand J, et al. The effect of drotrecogin alfa (activated) on long-term survival after severe sepsis. Crit Care Med 2004;32(11): 2199–206.

[22] Fourrier F. Recombinant human activated protein C in the treatment of severe sepsis: an evidence-based review. Crit Care Med 2004;31(11):S534–41.

[23] Zimmerman J. Use of blood products in sepsis: an evidence-based review. Crit Care Med 2004;32(11): S542–7.

[24] Manthous C. ARDS redux. Clinical Pulmonary Medicine 2006;13(2):121–7.

[25] Fenstermacher D, Hong Dennis. Mechanical ventilation: what have we learned? Crit Care Nurs Q 2004;27(3):258–94.

[26] Vender J, Szokol J, Murphy G, et al. Sedation, analgesia, and neuromuscular blockade in sepsis: an evidence-based review. Crit Care Med 2004;32(11): S554–61.

[27] Van den Berge G. Insulin therapy in critical illness. Canadian Journal of Diabetes 2004;28(1):43–9.

[28] Cariou A, Vinsonneau C, Dhainaut J. Adjunctive therapies in sepsis: an evidence-based review. Crit Care Med 2004;32(11):S562–70.

[29] Trzeciak S, Dellinger RP. Other supportive therapies in sepsis: an evidence- based review. Crit Care Med 2004;32(11) S751–7.

[30] Ferri F, Kuter D, Rao D. Disseminated intravascular coagulation. Available at: www.firstconsult.com. Accessed July 30, 2006.

CRITICAL CARE
NURSING CLINICS
OF NORTH AMERICA

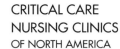

Crit Care Nurs Clin N Am 19 (2007) 87–97

Making Sense of Multiple Organ Dysfunction Syndrome

Stephen D. Krau, PhD, RN, CT

*Vanderbilt University Medical Center, School of Nursing, 314 Godchaux Hall,
21st Ave. South, Nashville, TN 37240, USA*

Despite the many advances in treating shock, renal failure, respiratory failure, and heart failure over the last few decades, the problem of multiple organ dysfunction syndrome (MODS) remains a major cause of death for patients in critical care areas. It is an entity that follows Osler's notion: patients usually die of complications of their disease rather than from the disease itself [1]. MODS has historically been the final complication of a critical illness, and accounts for the majority of deaths in noncoronary care units in the United States, with mortality rates well over 50% [2,3]. Some estimates of the mortality from MODS are as high as 70% [4]. MODS occurs when two or more organs are dysfunctional; however, when three or more organs are affected for more than 7 days, MODS carries a mortality of 60% to 98% [5]. Over 30 years after its initial description, the mortality of MODS remains unchanged, and is still the principle cause of morbidity and mortality for patients admitted to an intensive care unit, and the costs of treatment are colossal [6–8].

Definition of multiple organ dysfunction syndrome

Originally the syndrome we currently identify as MODS was called multiple organ failure. This terminology conveys a sense of inherent futility and a dichotomy of function versus failure, whereas in reality, there are relative levels of function of the organs involved in MODS. In the early 1970s, the syndrome was thought solely to be the result of an infection or sepsis [9]. In the

1980s, clinicians and researchers realized that infection was not inherently an antecedent to organ failure, and began to examine other processes that would explain the physiologic occurrences that resulted in organ dysfunction [10]. The lack of organ failure, and the progression of organ dysfunction toward failure resulted in the terminology "multiple organ system dysfunction" [9].

The American College of Chest Physicians (ACCP) and the Society of Critical Care Medicine (SCCM) [11] continue to address the issue of nomenclature among types of sepsis, systemic inflammation response syndrome (SIRS), and MODS. The results of their efforts is development of the definition of MODS, as indicated in Fig. 1.

MODS is the result of the immune system's response to a precipitating event. These events could include infection, sepsis, trauma, surgery, and any other event that assaults the integrity of the human body. Nomenclature of MODS includes *primary* MODS and *secondary* MODS. With the event of primary MODS, there is an initial insult or injury that is readily identified. This initial assault activates the immune system, particularly macrophages and neutrophils. Cytokines at this time alert the neutrophils and macrophages so they are ready to activate with any physiologic change [10,12].

Secondary MODS occurs days after the initial insult, and affects organs distant to the site of the initial injury. This response can be triggered by a minor physiologic insult because the body is already compromised. This phenomenon occurs because the cytokines are primed and ready to activate due to the initial assault [12]. In some cases, the difference between primary and secondary MODS is the timing of occurrence in the first week of hospital admission. Secondary MODS

E-mail address: stephen.krau@vanderbilt.edu

Definition of MODS from ACCP and SCCM
"Presence of altered organ function in an acutely ill person such that homeostasis, cannot be maintained with intervention. Primary MODS is the direct result of a well-defined insult in which organ dysfunction occurs early and [can] be directly attributable to the insult itself. Seconday MODS develops as a consequence of a host response and is identified within the context of SIRS (systemic inflammatory response syndrome)."
From American College of Chest Physicians/Society of Critical Care Medicine Consensus Conference Committee. (1992). Definitions for sepsis and organ failure and guidelines for the use of innovative therapies in sepsis. *Critical Care Medicine, 20,* 864-870.

Fig. 1. Definition of MODS.

often occurs in the context of SIRS, as identified by the ACCP/SCCM Consensus Conference Committee [13].

Systemic inflammation response syndrome

SIRS provides a context for MODS as the systemic inflammatory response can be triggered by a variety of assaulting conditions that can be either infectious or noninfectious. In situations where there is infection and a systemic inflammatory response, the patient is considered to be septic. However, it is important to note that signs of systemic inflammation can and do occur in the absence of infection [14]. A scheme of this context is shown in Fig. 2. This figure demonstrates the development of secondary MODS from Primary MODS. This scheme shows uncontrolled systemic inflammatory/stress response as a part of the processes in the development of secondary MODS. The processes are very dynamic, and vary in degree of severity from patient to patient.

Although SIRS is generally accepted as component or context in the pathogenesis of MODS, its measurement and quantification have remained elusive. Recognizing that infectious and noninfectious insults can result in similar responses, the American College of Chest Physicians, SCCM, the European Society of Intensive Care Medicine, the ACCP, the American Thoracic Society, and the Surgical Infection Society revised earlier diagnostic criteria for SIRS. The current criteria is in Box 1.

SIRS is the clinical consequence of systemic activation of the human inflammatory cascade. It is commonly the result of an invasive infection, but can be the result of shock, trauma, and burn injuries, and aseptic inflammation such as pancreatitis. When this mechanism overwhelms the critical threshold, defective oxygenation occurs

[15]. The inability of the host to use available oxygen to its benefit becomes the defining factor between SIRS and MODS. Failure to control the sustaining activation of SIRS and failure of the host to activate counterinflammatory measures leads to the progressive loss of organ function, and ultimately to the death of the patient [16].

Risk factors for the development of multiple organ dysfunction syndrome

The rationale that two people can endure the same initial insult and only one develop MODS is not completely clear. There are factors that predispose persons to an increase risk of developing MODS. These factors are an important component in the care of critical care patients so that nurses can identify persons who are at risk for the development of MODS.

These persons include are identified in Box 2.

Infection as a stimulus of MODS has been found to occur only half of the patients seen with MODS, whereas the other half demonstrate no clinically identifiable infectious etiology [17]. Thus, the patients who are diagnosed with MODS are a very heterogeneous population, which not only makes the pathogenesis of the syndrome complex, but also interventions, and research related to the syndrome [18]. Recently it was proposed that an autonomic dysfunction that is a feature of impaired organ communication might facilitate the development of MODS [19]. A basic feature in a normal functioning human body is the continuous communication between all vital organs through the autonomic nervous system. Autonomic dysfunction can contribute to severe inflammation. The result can be seen as SIRS, and other disturbances of the neurally mediated organ interactions and communications may lead to the development of MODS.

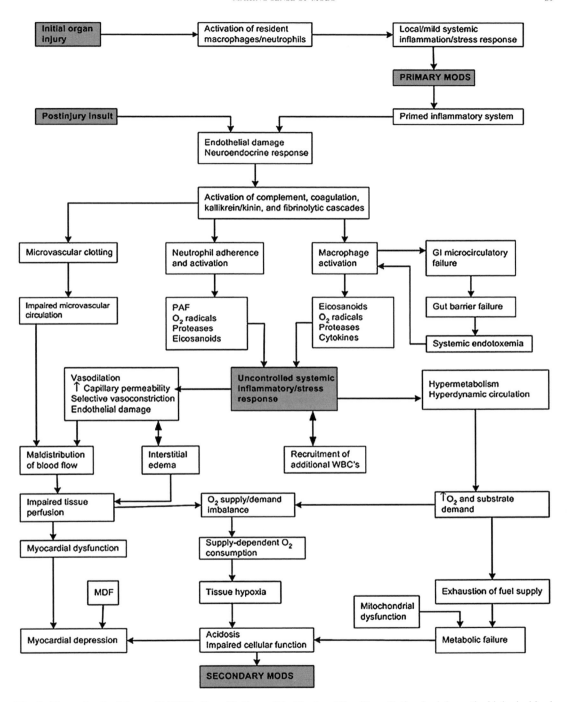

Fig. 2. The pathophysiology of MODS. *From* McCance KL, Huether SE, editors. Pathophysiology: the biological basis for disease in adults and children. 4th edition. Philadelphia: WB Saunders; 2002.

Box 1. American College of Chest Physicians (AACP), Society of Critical Care Medicine (SCCM), The European Society of Intensive Care Medicine (ESICM), the American Thoracic Society (ATS), and the Surgical Infection Society (SIS) Diagnostic Criteria for SIRS 2001

Diagnostic criteria for SIRS includes two or more of the following:
Body temperature >38°C or <36°C [14]
Tachycardia with heart rate >90 beats per minute [14]
Tachypnea manifested by respiratory rate >20 breaths per minute or $PaCO_2$ <32 mm Hg [14]
Leukocytosis or white blood cell count >12,000 cells/mm^3 or <4000 cells/mm^3 [14] or significant immature neutrophils (>10%) [9]

In 2001, the AACP, SCCM, American Thoracic Society, and European Society of Intensive Care Medicine updated the previous criteria to include the following:
Chills, decreased urine output, decreased skin perfusion hypoglycemia
Poor capillary refill petechiae, decreased platelet count skin mottling
Unexplained changes in mental status

Box 2. Persons at risk for development of MODS

Patients who have pancreatitis
Persons of advanced age
Trauma patients
Burn victims
Patients who have severe infections
Persons prone to chronic recurring infections
Patients who have experienced an aspiration
Multiple blood transfusion (>6 U in 12 h)
Patients who have chronic disease
Patients who have diabetes
Patients who have cancer
Renal insufficiency
Patients on immunosuppressant therapies
Patients who have been resuscitated but experience prolonged tissue hypoxia
Transplant patients
Patients who have pulmonary contusions
Patients experiencing conditions of endotoxin release
Shock patients
Patients who have widespread necrosis
Reperfusion following ischemia
Patients experiencing bowel infarction
Patients who have chronic alcoholism
Patients suffering from malnutrition
Patients with large hematomas

Theoretic basis for multiple organ dysfunction syndrome

As the basis for SIRS and MODS is complex, there are many theoretic etiologies that have been postulated. The major theories are presented in Table 1 [20–30].

Although one predominant theory has not been shown to be the single cause of SIRS or MODS, when combined, they offer a more complete explanation and plausible basis for MODS. Each theoretic base offers an explanation for MODS, and through understanding these theories, the rationale for interventions to ameliorate or prevent MODS become apparent to the critical care nurse. Whereas the multiple model approach may seem quite confusing, there is a need for more research to understand the mechanism underlying

these models individually and as a collective. Presenting these models in understandable terms and concepts is an important aspect of comprehending the mechanisms of MODS.

Making more sense of multiple organ dysfunction syndrome

Many clinicians view MODS as a consequence of the advances that have been made in modern medical care, and the ability to improve and prolong survival in persons with highly lethal disease processes and injuries. Before the advent of the advances made in the last 30 years, these patients would have most certainly died as a result of pathology we currently call "MODS."

Regardless of whether or not the catalyst is infection, the immune system and stress response, the body's own defense mechanisms, contribute to organs being compromised and ultimately failing [31]. The human immune system triggers events that respond in an effort to protect and defend the host and restore balance. The mediators that are released during the two main primary events of inflammatory/immune response (IIR), and neuroendocrine activity, initially serve the host as a defense and repair mechanism. However, the body loses the regulation of these functions, which results in a pathologic inundation of many inflammatory mediators. Responses that were initially localized become systemic derangements exacerbated by not only endothelial damage, but also ischemia/reperfusion injury [32].

To illustrate this point, vasodilation that occurs at the initial site of insult is the result of kinin and complement activity that could occur systematically. This could prompt systemic vasodilation, with the result being severe hypotension. Mediators that cause increased capillary permeability can upset the body fluid system by allowing the leakage of intravascular fluids into the interstium. This results in pulmonary edema, generalized edema, and severe hypotension.

The coagulation system is activated by tumor necrosis factor alpha (TNF-α) and interleukin 1, which stimulate the release of tissue factor which initiates the extrinsic coagulation pathway [33]. This activates the mechanism by which microemboli are formed and lodge in capillaries throughout the body. This, along with the already decreasing circulation due to the fluid shift, results in global tissue hypoxia [34].

When hypoxia occurs, the sympathetic nervous system mechanisms are activated to preserve bodily functions. This is commonly referred to as the "stress response" [16,31]. This mechanism actually compounds the problem, and results in further organ dysfunction. When the stress response is activated, adrenalin and epinephrine increase the rate of the heart and also activate to shunt more blood back to the heart. This, along with diminished circulating volume, deprives other organs of oxygen, particularly the gut and kidneys [31].

At this juncture the gut failure theory becomes of great consequence. Deitch and colleagues [29] maintain that after hemorrhagic shock, trauma, or burn injury, the gut released pro-inflammatory and tissue injurious factors can result in acute lung injury, bone marrow failure, myocardial dysfunction, neutrophil activation, red blood cell (RBC) injury, and endothelial cell activation and injury. This notion actually expands the mechanism of the gut in the process of MODS far beyond the "bacterial translocation" notion.

With the shunting of blood in the stress response, the kidneys are further deprived of perfusion. This not only impairs the ability of the kidneys to remove toxins from the body, but also makes their function as an acid-base buffer system ineffective. The hypoxia that is ensuing causes the body to become acidotic because it starts to use anaerobic metabolism to generate energy. With lactate being a major by-product of anaerobic metabolism, and the kidney buffer system impaired, lactic acidosis readily ensues. The lactate levels further exacerbate MODS by altering intracellular ion transport pumps and disrupt mitochondrial functions and normal carbohydrate metabolism [9]. In addition to the lactate acid disruption of normal carbohydrate metabolism, stress hormones block inflammation and put more of a demand on the body's energy needs by producing more circulating glucose [34,35]. The effect of this can further exacerbate the patient's problems by causing the retention of sodium and water, hyperglycemia, insulin resistance, and stress induced ulcers [35].

The respiratory buffer system in MODS is most likely already impaired, enhancing acidosis. Lungs are particularly sensitive to mediator-induced inflammation, and as such, are most often the first organs to show signs of failure in the progression of SIRS to MODS [34,36]. In addition, because of the fluid shift that has already occurred, the patient is most likely experiencing pulmonary edema, which further inhibits effective oxygenation during the highest points of demand.

A study by Schmidt and colleagues [37] suggests that the autonomic dysfunction associated with MODS disturbs the cardiorespiratory system. The study concludes that the more severe the MODS, the more the heart and lung coupling become impaired regardless of the age of the patient.

A paradox with MODS is the notion of "reperfusion injury." This is an occurrence in which hypoperfusion is corrected, and due to the blood flow to damaged cells, the cells that could be functional are progressively destroyed. When the immune system becomes disrupted, there is an outpouring of immature cells. The overproduction of histamine and bradykin, along with other complications and issues results in a systemic vasodilation that decreases systemic vascular resistance [38]. Consequently, distal end organs become further hypoperfused.

Table 1
Theoretical models and postulates of the etiology of MODS

Proposed pathologic process	Explanation of process
Uncontrolled infection	Although infection is not always a part of MODS [12], infection can be a part of this process. In some cases it is believed that the uncontrolled infection could be the result of the trigger event rather than the precipitating event of MODS. The earliest explanations of MODS contained strong correlations with infections [7]. Nosocomial infections were often attributed to be the etiology of MODS. Microbial products such as endotoxins may also cause MODS. Endotoxemia is much more common in critically ill patients than is documented infection [20]. This suggests the absorption of endotoxin from the gastrointestinal tract or lung as a cause of MODS [21].
Systemic inflammation with activation of cytokines	Clinical evidence of systemic inflammation is evident in a great majority of patients developing MODS [7,17]. Cytokines control many immune and inflammatory responses. Some cytokines are "pleiotropic" in that they affect many components of the immune system once activated. Other cytokines have specific actions. Although interleukins are the largest group of cytokines, interferons, colony stimulating factors, and tumor necrosis factors also activate to inflammation [22].
Microvascular coagulopathy	The complex interactions between coagulation and inflammation support the development and use of strategies that are aimed at improving endothelial cell function; an interruption in this process can increase the incidence of sepsis and MODS because the body is unable to modulate inflammation and coagulopathy [3]. When the balance of factors that balance the between coagulation and fibrinolysis, which commonly occurs in critical care patients, there is a shift toward a procoagulant state [7]. This shift usually precedes the development of organ dysfunction [24] and persists in those patients as they develop more dysfunction, or die [25].
Tissue hypoxia	Reduced or inadequate oxygen delivery or use inhibits normal physiologic processes, and as such, would be considered a pathway for MODS. Even in cases of successful resuscitation, the result can result in regional hypoxia. Additionally, increasing levels of lactate are associated with poor outcomes and suggestive of tissue hypoxia systemically or locally. Tissue hypoxia can also be the result of derangements in the cellular use of oxygen even in the presence of adequate oxygen. This phenomenon is called "cytopathic hypoxia" [7,26]. This can also be related to mitochondrial dysfunction [27].
Dysregulated apoptosis (premature cell death)	Apoptosis is a gene-directed method by which cells destruct. In normal physiologic conditions, it contributes to an orderly turnover of cells in all tissues [5]. Activation of the affector and effector systems, hormone release, and the cascade associated with cytokines are all components of the systemic process associated with SIRS and MODS. MODS-associated release of cytokines, interlueukin 1, and interleukin 6, as well as tumor necrosis factor (TNF) heat-shock proteins, oxidants, and glucocoricoids alters the rate of tissue apoptosis [7,28]. Although the mechanism of apoptosis in MODS is not clearly understood, an accelerated cell death of cells associated with immunity might ameliorate infection. Additionally, an accelerated rate may not only contribute to organ dysfunction or death, but in contrast, may be necessary for the resolution of inflammatory states. The timing of apoptosis and the cells involved are the main factors that determine whether the apoptosis will be beneficial or harmful to the patient [7]. A recent study by Knotzer and colleagues [27] supports numerous other studies that mitochondrial dysfunction leading to cytopathic hypoxia or increased apoptosis is a significant determinant in the severity and duration of MODS.

(continued on next page)

Table 1 (*continued*)

Proposed pathologic process	Explanation of process
Gut–liver axis-mediated infections	The "gut hypothesis" of MODS has undergone multiple changes during the last several decades, and has evolved from the concept of bacterial translocation being the dominant factor. The normal human gut has millions of endotoxins and bacteria that outside of the gastrointestinal tract could easily kill the host. Even small increases in gut permeability and "bacterial translocation" would have profound consequences [29]. With gut-origin MODS, it is thought that gut ischemia and loss of barrier function lead to the host-producing endogenous proinflammatory and tissue injurious factors that lead to organ injury. In fact, gut ischemia appears to be the dominant link by which splanchnic hypoperfusion is transduced from a hemodynamic event into an immunoinflammatory event via the release of biologically active factors into the mesenteric lymphatics [29,30].

Therapeutic management of patients with multiple organ dysfunction syndrome

As MODS is a complex process, the therapeutic management for each patient may vary depending on the risk factors of the patient and the organs involved. The management of MODS remains difficult, and there continues to be controversy over interventions, but the goals of management are all inclusive for MODS. These goals include (a) prevention, (b) identifying risk factors, (c) control infectious or inflammatory stimuli, (d) balancing oxygen supply and demand, (e) provide nutritional support to meet metabolic requirements, and (f) individual organ support [9,38,39].

Prevention

The most salient aspect of treatment for any patient at risk for the development of sepsis, SIRS, or MODS is prevention [40]. A complete and thorough history is key to prevention or exacerbation of the spiral from the initial insult to MODS. In addition, all treatable injuries at time of admission need to be addressed immediately, as the patient is closely monitored. Fractures should be set; and if surgery is indicated for the presenting problem, it should be done quickly. Once initiated, the systemic IIR fulminates with even minimal exogenous stimuli even after the initial insult is addressed [39].

Identification of risk factors

Any patient admitted to the intensive care unit has the potential for developing sepsis that can spiral to MODS. Those patients at particular risk should be monitored closely due to their vulnerability. There are special considerations for different

risks, and although the mechanisms related to these particular risks are not within the scope of this particular discussion, these considerations are important for the critical care nurse to recognize. Patients that are of particular risk have been identified in Box 2.

Control of infections of infectious stimuli

Early identification and control of infections and potential for infections is a salient goal in treating as well as contributing to the prevention of MODS. Infection control is a major component of prevention and treatment. With the high incidence iatrogenic infections that occur in intensive care units, this is of particular importance. Patients who are at risk for MODS should be closely monitored for signs of infections. Efforts toward eradicating the cause, once it is identified, with specific antibiotic administration is an important aspect of treatment. Even with the potential for strong organ toxicity, coverage for specific organisms merit specific antibiotic coverage immediately. In some cases, surgical debridement and/or incision and draining from abscesses may be warranted [40].

Intensive care units are still associated with a high incidence of nosocomial infections. Key nursing interventions for patients who are at risk for MODS center around monitoring. Vigilante observations of all lines, catheters, along with aggressive wound and skin care are essential. The other important issue that remains an ongoing challenge for even the best nurses is meticulous handwashing. Standard infection prevention protocols should be well enforced.

The use of corticosteroids to minimize inflammatory response has been the cause of much controversy. The overwhelming evidence supports that corticosteroids are not indicated in SIRS or MODS [39,41]. The side effects of corticosteroids, including the immunosuppression effect, is of particular concern in MODS patients. This effect actually predisposes the patient to greater complications [39,42,43]. Although low-dose hydrocortisone has been shown to suppress the immune system in some studies, it is not regarded as a conventional treatment. Currently there are studies in nonhumans that indicate the administration of granulocyte/macrophage colony-stimulating factors may be beneficial in the treatment of sepsis or secondary infection by enhancing and reconstituting the compromised immune system [44]. This treatment is experimental in many cases, but has been approved for other conditions such as severe chronic neutropenia, and bone marrow transplantation [44].

Tissue factor pathway inhibitor is a treatment that interrupts the clotting cascade. This interruption occurs both within the intrinsic and extrinsic pathways, and has potential for ameliorating the effects associated with coagulation effects of MODS. Anti-TNF antibody therapy also alters the inflammatory response [9].

Xigris, which is activated protein C, is medication that decreases inflammation and increases fibrinolysis, which helps with the microvascular complications associated with MODS. Additionally, patients who receive Xigris in several studies had a more rapid decline in interleukin-6 levels, a global marker of inflammation, consistent with a reduction in the inflammatory response. It is the only drug that has been shown to decrease the mortality in MODS [45,46].

A recent study by Cibrian and colleagues [47] indicates that the use of growth-hormone-releasing peptide-6 is effective in the use of visceral vascular hypoperfusion in rodents. The synthetic form is small and inexpensive. More studies are needed to conclude that patients who are at risk for MODS who are given growth-hormone-releasing peptide-6 as an early intervention have better chances of maintaining organ viability.

Balancing oxygen supply and demand

Oxygen transport formulas such as oxygen delivery and oxygen consumption provide the clinician with data more valuable than arterial saturation and cardiac output. Using formulas based on oxygen delivery and oxygen consumption reveal the how much oxygen the body is actually using, and is a stronger indicator of what is happening in the patient. These parameters help the clinician meet the goals of (a) optimizing oxygen supply, (b) reverse any oxygen debt that may have occurred, and (c) show which interventions help decrease oxygen demand. These three components provide the basis for balancing oxygen supply and demand.

Oxygen supply is enhanced through the use of vasopressors such as dopamine and epinephrine or norepinephrine, particularly in distal organs when vasodilation occurs. These drugs help increase systemic vascular resistance and work to make the patient normotensive. Improved survival rates have been shown in cases where supranormal values for cardiac index, oxygen delivery, and consumption were reached [40,48]. Volume resuscitation also impacts the supply and demand balance, and blood that has become thickened due to fluid shifts to the interstitial spaces flows more easily. Additionally, this enhances cardiac output to maintain intravascular volume and thus to optimize preload.

Decreasing oxygen demand

Because oxygen demand is greater than supply in patients with MODS, it is imperative to institute interventions that will decrease the oxygen demand. Any condition such as fever, chills, pain, tachycardia, and increased respirations increases demand on an already oxygen-deprived system. Interventions that reduce oxygen demand are as important as those increase oxygen supply. These symptoms need to be controlled so the patient, if not already, might be placed on a ventilator. In some patients, particularly the elderly, there is sometimes a hesitancy to initiate ventilator support because of the potential for ventilator dependence [40]. When the patient is on a ventilator, a plethora of ventilator issues and complications related to mechanical ventilation can actually lead to further systemic compromise. These warrant the attention of the nurse, including meticulous mouth care.

Excessive body temperatures need to be reduced with hypothermic blankets or devices, and controlled with medications such as acetaminophen. Optimizing pain medications and sedation increases comfort of the patient, and decreases oxygen demand. Medications aimed at decreasing pain and relaxing the patient also decrease heart oxygen demand, decrease the work of breathing, and decrease restlessness, all of which help decrease the oxygen demand. Analgesics also enhance toleration to invasive procedures, turning, suctioning, and line insertion, hence helping ameliorate oxygen demand.

Meeting metabolic demands through nutritional support

The same phenomena that increase the demand for oxygenation also tax the metabolic system, as the body continues to revert to catabolic mechanisms to meet its energy demands. Conserving oxygen overlaps with the importance of providing nutritional support to support metabolism. Early enteral and parenteral nutrition should be initiated. Delays in nutritional support result in hypermetabolism and muscle catabolism. These mechanisms further contribute to functional losses, and inhibit optimal recovery.

There is much controversy about which nutritional therapies are most effective under different circumstances; however, overwhelming evidence supports enteral feedings as opposed to total parenteral nutrition. Enteral feeding reduces complications and helps maintain the gut barrier function [40,49,50]. Total parenteral nutrition, which is usually given to allow bowel rest, actually contributes to atrophy of the intestinal mucosa, which may contribute "bacterial translocation" and endotoxemia. If full alimentation is not possible, small amounts of enteral nutrition should be initiated to maintain mucosal integrity [40]. In addition, enteral feedings decrease the incidence of stress ulceration, support hepatic function, enhance the immune system, and prevent bile sludging [51].

Support of individual organs

Although this is a major goal in the interventions for the patients with MODS, even the individual organs must be viewed in terms of the total disease process and removing the stimulus of IIR. Supportive care treats symptoms and manifestations, but it does not treat the underlying source of the problem.

The lungs are usually the first organs to show signs of dysfunction and impending failure in the progression from SIRS to MODS. In the event of acute respiratory distress syndrome, the patient should be placed on a ventilator. This not only supports the organ, but has obvious implications oxygen supply and demand.

Research has shown there is a decrease in heart rate variability in MODS as the result of sepsis [52]. Keep in mind that if coupling is broken,

which is referred to as *decomplexification,* that the communication between the heart and other organs becomes interrupted. In addition, when the pancreas is inadequately perfused for a prolonged period, it secretes a factor into the system that serves as a myocardial depressant to further compromise the efficacy of the heart [38].

The hypoperfused kidneys prevent the clearing of toxins, and eventually this leads to kidney failure. Support for the function of the kidneys might be achieved through dialysis. Liver enzymes are usually elevated as liver becomes dysfunctional, and the patient may become jaundiced. Be sure to watch ammonia levels and changes in sensorium if the patient is not sedated.

One organ that commonly gets ignored during MODS is the skin. The skin is one of the largest organs of the body, and like any other organ, can become dysfunctional and fail. The skin serves a vast variety of functions including protection, regulation of temperature, storage of fat and water, waste exchange, and vitamin D synthesis. As blood and nutrients are shunted, and the potential for edema increases due to the endothelial issues in MODS, the skin is vulnerable. Like any other organ that is in the process of failing, failing skin can contribute to the downward spiral of MODS as it becomes damaged and necrotic [53]. The integrity of the skin should be maintained through proper turning and special beds or bed equipment.

Most hospitals have measurement tools or scoring instruments to help determine the level of dysfunction. There are abundant tools such as the sequential organ failure assessment, the multiple organ dysfunction score, the acute physiology and chronic health evaluation, both forms, and the logistic organ dysfunction system, which are used to measure levels of organ dysfunction [38]. There are numerous other tools available to assess the extent of MODS. This sometimes impacts the ability to generalize discussion when comparing research studies because of different measurements have some variations. Nonetheless, a decrease in function of any organ is cause for concern, and when two or more become dysfunctional, the patient has multiple organ dysfunction syndrome.

Summary

Despite recent advances in critical care medicine, caring for patients with MODS remains one of the most challenging experience a critical care can encounter. New therapies that current exist and continue to be developed contribute to successful outcomes for patients with MODS, but there is no substitute for prevention and early intervention for persons at risk for developing MODS. Early and subtle changes in the patient who is at risk and has endured an initial insult can make a great difference in the patient's outcome and chances of mortality. Goal-directed therapy, supportive management, as well as an understanding of the inflammatory process are key to decreasing the mortality rates among patients with MODS.

References

[1] Beal AL, Cerr FB. Multiple organ failure syndrome in the 1990s: systemic inflammatory response and organ dysfunction. JAMA 1994;271(3):226–33.

[2] Faist E, Baue AE, Dittmer H, et al. Multiple organ failure in polytrauma patients. J Trauma 1983;118: 243–9.

[3] Pine RW, Wertz MJ, Lennard ES, et al. Determinants of organ malfunction or death in patients with intra-abdrominal sepsis: a discriminant analysis. Arch Surg 1983;118:243–9.

[4] Schmidt H, Muller-Werden U, Hoffman T, et al. Autonomic dysfunction predicts mortality in patient with multiple organ dysfunction syndrome in different age groups. Crit Care Med 2005;3(9):1994–2002.

[5] Lydon A, Jeevendra-Martin JA. Apoptosis in critical illness. Int Anesthesiol Clin 2003;41(1):65–77.

[6] Vollman TJ, Hendricks T, Gors RA. Zymosan-induced generalized inflammation: experimental studies into mechanisms leading to multiple organ dysfrunction syndrome. Shock 2005;23(4):291–7.

[7] Marshall JC. Inflammation, coagulopathy, and the pathogenesis of multiple organ dysfunction syndrome. Crit Care Med 2001;29:S99–S106.

[8] Angus DC, Linde-Zwirble WT, Lidicker J, et al. Epidemiology of severe sepsis in United States: analysis of incidence, outcome, and associated costs of care. Crit Care Med 2001;29:1303–10.

[9] Walsh CR. Multiple organ dysfunction syndrome after multiple trauma. Orthop Nurs 2005;24(5): 324–33.

[10] Walsh CR. Multiple organ dysfunction syndrome. In: Melander SD, editor. Case studies in critical care nursing: a guide for application and review. 3rd edition. Philadelphia: W.B. Saunders; 2004. p. 352–69.

[11] American College of Chest Physicians/Society of Critical Care Medicine Consensus Conference Committee. Definitions for sepsis and organ failure and guidelines for the use of innovative therapies in sepsis. Crit Care Med 1992;20:864–70.

[12] Baldwin KM, Morris SD. Shock, multiple organ dysfunction syndrome, and burns in adults and children. In: McCance KL, Huether SE, editors.

[13] Pathophysiology: the biological basis for disease in adults and children. 4th edition. Philadelphia: W.B. Saunders; 2002. p. 1483–512.

[13] Tantalean JA, Leon RJ, Santos AA, et al. Multiple organ dysfunction syndrome in children. Pediatr Crit Care Med 2003;4(2):181–5.

[14] Levy M, Fink M, Marshall J, et al. 2001 SCCM/ ESICM/ACCP/ATS/SIS International Sepsis Definitions Conditions. Crit Care Med 2003;31(4): 1250–6.

[15] Offner PJ, Moore EE. Risk factors for MOF and pattern of organ failure following severe trauma. In: Baue AE, Eugen F, Fry DE, editors. Mutiple organ failure: pathophysiology, prevention, and therapy. New York: Springer; 2000. p. 30–43.

[16] Fry DE. Systemic inflammation response and multiple organ dysfunction syndrome: biologic domino effect. In: Baue AE, Eugen F, Fry DE, editors. Mutiple organ failure: pathophysiology, prevention, and therapy. New York: Springer; 2000. p. 23–39.

[17] Marshall J, Sweeney D. Microbial infection and the septic response in critical surgical illness. Arch Surg 1990;125:17–23.

[18] Hoyer D, Friedrich H, Zweiner U, et al. Prognostic impact of autonomic information flow in multiple organ dysfunction syndrome patients. Int J Cardiol 2006;108:356–69.

[19] Moerer O, Schmid A, Hoffman M, et al. Direct costs of severe sepsis in three German intensive care units based on retrospective electronic patient record analysis of resource use. Intensive Care Med 2002; 28(10):1440–6.

[20] Danner RL, Elin RJ, Hosseini JM, et al. Endotoxemia in human septic shock. Chest 1991;99:169–75.

[21] Murphy DB, Cregg N, Tremblay L, et al. Adverse ventilatory strategy causes pulmonary-to-systemic translocation of endotoxin. Am J Respir Crit Care Med 2000;162:27–33.

[22] Workman ML. Concepts of inflammation and the immune response. In: Ignatavicius DD, Workman ML, editors. Medical-surgical nursing: critical thinking for collaborative care. 5th edition. St. Louis (MO): Elsevier; 2006. p. 360–79.

[23] Vincent JL. Microvascular endothelial dysfunction: a renewed appreciation of sepsis pathophysiology. Crit Care 2001;5(Suppl 2):S1–5.

[24] Leithauser B, Matthias FR, Nicolai U, et al. Hemostaticss abnormalities and the severity of illness in patients at the onset of clinically defined sepsis: possible indication of the degree of endothelial cell activation? Intensive Care Med 1996;22:631–6.

[25] Boldt J, Papsdorf M, Rothe A, et al. Changes of the hemostatic network in in critically ill patients: is there a difference between sepsis, trauma, and neurosurgery patients? Crit Care Med 2000;28:445–50.

[26] Dubin A, Murias G, Maskin B, et al. Increased blood flow prevents intramucosal acidosis in sheep endotoxemia: a controlled study. Crit Care 2005; 9(2):R66–73.

[27] Knotzer H, Pajk W, Dunser MW, et al. Regional microvascular function and vascular reactivity in patients with different degrees of multiple organ dysfunction syndrome. Anesth Analg 2006;102(4):1187–93.

[28] Papathanassoglou E, Moynihan J, Ackerman M. Does programmed cell death (apoptosis) play a role in the development of multiple organ dysfunction in critically ill patients? A review and a theoretical framework. Crit Care Med 2000;28:537–49.

[29] Deitch EA, Xu D, Kaise VL. Role of the gut in the development of injury- and shock induced SIRS and MODS: the gut-lymph hypothesis, a review. Front Biosci 2006;11:520–8.

[30] Magnotti Louis J, Deitch Edwin A. Burns, bacterial translocation, gut barrier function and failure. J Burn Care Rehabil 2005;26(5):383–91.

[31] Duhon JL. When organs fail one by one. RN 2006;69(5):44–7.

[32] Secor VH. Multiple organ dysfunction syndrome: background, etiology, and sequence of events. In: Secor VH, editor. Multiple organ dysfunction & failure: pathophysiology and clinical complications. 2nd edition. St. Louis (MO): Mosby; 1996. p. 3–18.

[33] Kleinpell R. Advances in treating patients with severe sepsis: role of drotrecogin alfa (activated). Crit Care Nurse 2003;3(3):16–24.

[34] Kaplan L. Systemic inflammatory response syndrome. 2004. Available at: http://www.emedicine.com/med/topic3372.htm. Accessed October 10, 2006.

[35] Kleinpell RM. Multisystem problems. In: Chulay M, Burns SM, editors. AACN essentials of critical care nursing. New York: McGraw-Hill; 2006. p. 267–78.

[36] Bhatia M, Moochhala S. Role of inflammatory mediators in pathophysiology of acute respiratory distress syndrome. J Pathol 2004;202(2):145–56.

[37] Schmidt H, Muller-Werden U, Nuding S, et al. Impaired chemoreflex sensitivity in adult patients with multiple organ dysfunction syndrome—the potential role of disease severity. Intensive Care Med 2004;30:665–72.

[38] Phillips RA. Stopping the train wreck of SIRS. Nursing Made Incredibly Easy. 2006; July/August:44–54.

[39] Secor VH. Multiple organ dysfunction syndrome: overview and conclusions. In: Secor VH, editor. Multiple organ dysfunction & failure: pathophysiology and clinical complications. 2nd edition. St. Louis (MO): Mosby; 1996. p. 402–23.

[40] Rauen CA, Stamatos CA. Caring for geriatric patients with MODS. Am J Nurs 1997;97(5):16BB–HH.

[41] Nicholson DP. Review of corticosteroid treatment in sepsis and septic shock: pro or con. Crit Care Clin 1989;5:151–5.

[42] Bernard GR, et al. High-dose corticosteroids in patients with adult respiratory distress syndrome. N Engl J Med 1987;317:1565–70.

[43] Boone RC, Fisher CJ Jr, Clemmer TP, et al. A controlled clinical trial of high-dose methylprednisolone in the treatment of severe sepsis and septic shock. N Engl J Med 1987;317:653–8.

[44] Hartung T, von Aulock S, Albrecht W. Growth factors G-CSF and GM-CSF: clinical options. In: Baue AE, Faist E, Fry DE, editors. Multiple organ failure: pathophysiology, prevention, and therapy. New York: Springer-Verlag; 2000. p. 621–9.

[45] Manns BJ, Lee H, Doig CJ, et al. An economic evaluation of activated protein C treatment for severe sepsis. N Engl J Med 2002;347:993–1000.

[46] Peck P (2004). Early initiation of drotrecogin alpha may improve survival. Medscape Medical News. Available at: http://www.medscape.com/viewarticle/470592. Accessed September, 2006.

[47] Cibrian D, Ajamieh H, Berlanga J, et al. Use of growth-hormone-releasing peptide-6 (GHRP-6) for the prevention of multiple organ failure. Clin Sci 2006;110:563–73.

[48] Shoemaker WC, Appel PL, Kram HB, et al. Hemodynamic and oxygen transport monitoring to titrate therapy in septic shock. New Horiz 1993;1:145–59.

[49] Deitch EA. The role of intestinal barrier failure and bacterial translocation in the development of systemic infection and multiple organ failure. Arch Surg 1990;125:403–4.

[50] Alexander JW. Immunoenhancement via enteral nutrition. Arch Surg 1993;128:1242–5.

[51] Rivers E, Nguyen B, Havstad S, et al. Early goal directed therapy in the treatment of severe sepsis and septic shock. N Engl J Med 2001;345(19):1368–77.

[52] Pontet J, Contreras P, Curbelo J, et al. Heart rate variability as early marker of multiple organ dysfunction syndrome in septic patients. J Crit Care 2003;18(3):156–63.

[53] Langemo DK, Brown G. Skin fails too: acute, chronic and end-stage skin failure. Adv Wound Care 2006;19(4):206–11.

CRITICAL CARE
NURSING CLINICS
OF NORTH AMERICA

Crit Care Nurs Clin N Am 19 (2007) 99–106

Managing the Infected Heart

Maria A. Smith, DSN, RN, CCRN, COI[a],*, Tasha L. Smith, BA[b],
Beth Towery Davidson, MSN, RN, ACNP, CCRN[c]

[a]School of Nursing, Middle Tennessee State University, 1500 Greenland Drive, P.O. Box 81, Murfreesboro,
TN 37132, USA
[b]Tennessee Cardiovascular Research Institute (A Division of The Heart Group, PLLC), 4230 Harding Road,
Suite 330, Nashville, TN 37205, USA
[c]The Heart Group, 4230 Harding Road, Suite 330, Nashville, TN 37205, USA

Infective endocarditis (IE) is a devastating infection of cardiac tissue that affects individuals on a global scale. Since this disease was recognized 450 years ago, diagnosis and treatment have continued to challenge health care professionals. The incidence of IE is 1.4 to 4.2 per 100,000 persons diagnosed annually in the United States. Despite advances in microbiologic identification and treatment, IE still has a high mortality rate of 21% to 35% [1].

Conditions associated with IE include injection-drug use, body piercing, poor dental hygiene, mechanical valves, long-term hemodialysis, and implantable pacemakers and cardioverter-defibrillators. IE can affect the endocardium, cardiac chambers, septum, and valves. Valvular structures are the most commonly affected. These structural cardiovascular dysfunctions lead to valvular insufficiency, congestive heart failure (CHF), and myocardial abscesses.

Acute and subacute infective endocarditis

IE may be acute or subacute in presentation. Acute IE has a rapid onset and short incubation period that may be days to weeks. The cause of acute IE is usually an aggressive virulent bacterium such as *Staphylococcus aureus*. Patients usually present with severe symptoms, and their overall health status can decline quickly because of bacterial virulence. Damage to cardiac structures will result in death without prompt diagnosis and initiation of aggressive management.

Subacute IE is more gradual in onset and represents long-standing incubation. The cause of subacute IE is usually a less virulent bacterium such as *Streptococcus viridans*. Symptoms present over weeks to months, and the patient presents with less dramatic clinical symptoms. Subacute IE can occur in individuals who have preexisting cardiac defects.

Pathogenesis

Intact endocardial tissue is virtually impermeable to bacterial invasion, but defects in endocardial tissue provide an opportunity for IE to develop. Endocardial defects can occur from congenital or acquired cardiac mechanisms. These defects serve as reservoirs for fibrin and platelet aggregation. The initial sterile vegetations that form serve as the foundation for bacterial colonization. Proliferation of bacteria and platelet and fibrin aggregation increase and produce enlarged vegetative growth. These areas of vegetation can break off, producing free-floating septic emboli that can lodge in various body organs (ie, brain, kidneys, spleen) and affect multiple systems (ie, respiratory, cardiovascular, integumentary, gastrointestinal, and neuromuscular).

When a defect occurs in the endocardium, IE can result from one of two mechanisms. The first mechanism is direct infection by virulent microorganisms. Bacteria in the circulating bloodstream attach to the injury site and produce IE. A second

* Corresponding author.
  E-mail address: massmith@mtsu.edu (M.A. Smith).

mechanism starts with a vegetative mass of fibrin and platelets that adheres to the injury site and produce a nonbacterial thrombotic endocarditis. Bacteria invade and colonize on the thrombotic mass resulting in IE.

Pathogens in infective endocarditis

IE can be community or hospital acquired. Although bacterial invasion causes most IE, fungi also can be a source of this disease. Major bacterial causes of IE include staphylococci, streptococci, and enterococci. IE can be caused by coagulase-positive staphylococci (*Staphylococcus aureus*) or coagulase-negative staphylococci (*Staphylococcus epidermis* and other species). Traditional thinking considered coagulase-positive staphylococci as the causative factor only for native valve endocarditis and coagulase-negative staphylococci to be the causative factor for prosthetic valve endocarditis, but current research does not support this hypothesis. Research has shown that prosthetic valve and native valve endocarditis can result from both pathogens [2].

Globally, *Staphylococcus aureus* is the most common cause of IE [3]. This can be attributed to lifestyle and longevity. Injection drug use precipitates *Staphylococcus aureus* IE involving the right side of the heart, specifically the tricuspid valve. It has a greater than 85% cure rate with short-course pharmaceutical treatment. This disease is most prevalent in younger persons. Longer lifespan increases the probability of contact with health care systems. In older individuals this contact results in surgical and procedural interventions , such as placement of prosthetic valves for degenerative valve disease. These interventions can expose the individual to *Staphylococcus aureus*. In persons who do not use injection drugs, IE predominantly involves the left side of the heart and has a 25% to 40% mortality rate [4]. The incidence of this disease is greater in the older population.

Community-acquired native IE in persons who do not use intravenous drugs has been linked to *Streptococci viridans* or α-hemolytic streptococci as causative agents. Although species such as *Streptococcus sanguis*, *Streptococcus oralis*, *Streptococcus salivarius*, and *Streptococcus mutans* are among the most common causative agents, other viridans groups that cause IE are *Abiotrophia defective*, *Granulicatella* species, and *Gemella* species.

HACEK group microorganisms account for 5% to 10% of IE cases. (The acronym "HACEK" refers to the following group of gram-negative bacilli: *Haemophilus parainfluenza*, *H aphrophilus*, *H paraphrophilus*, *H influenza*, *Actinobacillas actinomycetemcomitans*, *Cardiobacteriuhominis*, *Eikenella corrodens*, *Kingella kingae*, and *K aenitrificans*.) These organisms produce endocardial infections involving native valves and are the most common cause of gram-negative endocarditis among persons who are not intravenous drug abusers.

Fungal endocarditis results from *Candida* and *Aspergillus* species, with *Candida* being the most common cause. Patients who have fungal endocarditis often have multiple predisposing conditions such as prosthetic valves and central invasive catheters. Fungal endocarditis can be a complication of these surgical procedures.

Diagnosing fungal endocarditis is challenging because of its response to attempted laboratory culture. Blood cultures that generally are used to facilitate pathogen identification present a negative finding in *Aspergillus*-related fungal endocarditis. *Candida*-related endocarditis produces a positive laboratory culture, which aids in pathogen identification.

These identified pathogens are not the only causes of IE. There are increasing reports of new bacterial species (eg, *Tropheryma whipplei* and *Bartonella* species) and uncommon organisms (eg, *Finegoldia* species, *Gemella* species, and *Abiotrophia defective*) causing IE [1]. As antibiotic resistance increases, new bacterial strains will appear.

Clinical presentation

Fever is the most common sign and symptom in IE. Care must be taken to assess other manifestations, because fever can be reduced or absent in patients suffering from severe debility, chronic renal failure, or CHF. Symptoms can involve the respiratory, integumentary, gastrointestinal, cardiac, and neuromuscular systems in addition to generalized nonspecific complaints. Because symptoms are often flulike, patients may seek relief with antibiotic therapy, which can mask fever originating from other bacterial sources (Table 1).

Diagnosis

Diagnosis of IE requires integration of clinical, laboratory, and echocardiographic data. Nonspecific findings, such as anemia, leukocytosis,

Table 1
Signs and symptoms of infective endocarditis

System	Presentation
Respiratory	Shortness of breath
Cardiovascular	Murmur
	Congestive heart failure
Integumentary	Painless, flat, erythematous, hemorrhagic/pustule lesions on palms or soles (Janeway lesions)
	Splinter hemorrhages under the fingernails or toenails
	Tender subcutaneous nodules on the pulps of the fingers or toes (Osler's nodes)
	Round white spots surrounded by hemorrhage in the retina (Roths spots)
	Petechia on the skin, conjunctiva, and/or oral mucosa
Gastrointestinal	Poor appetite
	Anorexia
Neuromuscular	Arthralgia
	Joint pain
	Headache
	Altered sensorium
	Cranial nerve defects (eg, hemianopsia)
General	Fatigue
	Low-grade fever
	Chills
	Night sweats
	Anemia
	Weight loss
	Splenomegaly

elevated erythrocyte sedimentation rate, and elevated C-reactive protein, may be present [5].

Laboratory data

The standard for diagnosing IE is the documentation of bacteremia based on blood culture results. Because endocarditis is characterized by persistent bacteremia over time, several sets of positive cultures should be obtained at different sites and times before the initiation of antibiotics [6].

Imaging studies

Although blood cultures remain central in the diagnosis of IE, echocardiography is the indirect diagnostic method of choice [7]. Both transthoracic and transesophageal echocardiography have indications for use (Box 1).

A positive echocardiogram for IE is defined as an oscillating intracardiac mass on a valve or other supporting structure, in the path of regurgitant jets or on implanted material in the absence of other alternative explanation, an abscess or fistula, or a new parital dehiscence of valve prosthesis [8]. Other imaging studies that may be indicated based on the differential diagnoses include electrocardiography, chest radiograph, and chest and head CT.

Duke criteria for infective endocarditis

In 1994, a group at Duke University proposed standardized criteria for assessment of patients suspected of having IE. These criteria used major and minor classifications to facilitate diagnosis. They integrated predisposing factors, blood-culture results, echocardiographic findings, and other clinical and laboratory data.

Major criteria include two categories relevant to positive blood cultures for IE and evidence of endocardial involvement that includes a positive echocardiogram or new valvular regurgitation. The six minor criteria are (1) predisposition to cardiac involvement; (2) fever in excess of 38°C or 100.4°F; (3) vascular phenomena that include arterial emboli, pulmonary infarction, intracranial and conjunctival hemorrhage, and Janeway lesions; (4) immunologic phenomena that include Osler's nodes, Roth spots, glomerulonephritis, and rheumatoid factor; (5) microbiologic evidence

---

Box 1. Indications for the use of transthoracic echocardiography and transesophageal echocardiography

Transthoracic echocardiography
Good quality images
Low clinical suspicion of IE involving native valve

Transesophageal echocardiography
Negative transthoracic echocardiography study
High clinical suspicion of IE involving native or prosthetic valve
Positive transthoracic echocardiography and complications likely
Before cardiac surgery during active IE

of positive blood cultures or serologic evidence of an active infection; and (6) echocardiographic evidence of IE not consistent with major criterion findings.

Pathologic criteria include microorganisms (culture or histology) and/or pathologic lesions (vegetation, abscess, or fistula). Clinical assessment criteria are the presence of two major criteria, or one major and three minor criteria, or five minor criteria [9].

Complications

Congestive heart failure

The development of CHF in IE is valve dependent. CHF occurs more frequently in patients who have aortic valve infections than in those who have mitral or tricuspid valve infections [10]. In addition, tolerance to the valve dysfunction that results from IE differs based on left- or right-sided valve involvement. Dysfunction of the tricuspid valve, on the low-pressure right side of the heart, is better tolerated than dysfunction of the aortic valve on the high-pressure left side of the heart.

The degree of CHF depends on the amount of dysfunction and the valve involved. CHF may be acute or insidious in onset. Acute CHF may result from abrupt valve dysfunction resulting from chordae tendinae rupture, obstruction of valves by vegetative masses, sudden intracardiac shunts caused by fistula development, or valve leaflet perforation. Insidious CHF in IE can result despite antibiotic intervention. Close monitoring is imperative to identify changes in heart sounds and hemodynamic changes refractory to treatment, which may indicate IE-induced CHF.

CHF in patients who have IE negatively affects the overall prognosis [10]. Patients who experience CHF have poorer long-term outcomes. Echocardiographic evaluation can assist in early identification and prompt intervention. Surgery, such as valve replacement or repair, may be required to break the cycle of refractory CHF resulting from IE.

Periannular infection

Anatomically, annular tissue near the septum and the atrioventricular node is weaker than other myocardial tissue. When annular infections extend into this tissue, perivalvular cavities form. Periannular infection is associated with CHF and a higher mortality rate. Atrioventricular node involvement can result in heart block [11].

Periannular infection occurs in 10% to 40% of native valve IE. Valvular involvement varies. Extension beyond the valve annulus complicates aortic valve IE more often than IE involving the mitral or tricuspid valves. Prosthetic valve IE is more common than native valve IE because the annulus, rather than the valve leaflet, emerges as the primary infection site [12].

Because of cardiovascular pressure, abscesses may progress to fistulas that can create intracardiac shunts. A mortality rate of 40% has been reported when shunts occur [13]. Mortality probability increases when infection as a result of shunting is complicated by CHF or in patients who have prosthetic valves.

Intervention includes aggressive antibiotic therapy and/or surgical intervention. Antibiotic therapy usually is more successful for smaller infectious lesions. Surgical intervention is the treatment of choice. Options for surgical intervention include valve replacement, removal of necrotic tissue resulting from IE, drainage of pus from abscesses, and fistula repair [14]. Following removal of infected and necrotic tissue and placement of a more competent valve, the patient should be more hemodynamically stable.

Splenic infarction/abscess

Embolized vegetation can detach and migrate to the splenic artery. There it can cause partial or total occlusion that compromises blood flow to the point of splenic infarction. Bacterial infiltration of the splenic tissue then can result in pus-filled cavities or abscesses, a common complication of left-sided IE.

Clinical signs and symptoms of splenic infarction and abscesses include back pain, left flank or upper quadrant pain, or abdominal tenderness [15]. Patients who have splenic infarction and abscess also demonstrate persistent fever [15] or persistent or recurrent positive blood cultures. Abdominal CT and MRI demonstrate contrast-enhancing cystic lesions. Treatment is aimed at reducing the bacterial contents of the cyst by percutaneous drainage or total removal of the infected spleen (laparoscopic or open abdominal splenectomy). Untreated splenic abscesses are fatal [16]. Lack of consensus regarding treatment can result in variable approaches to the management and resolution of splenic complications. Aggressive antibiotic therapy should continue after the procedure.

Neurologic complications

Twenty percent to 40% of patients who have IE demonstrate neurologic complications [17]. Neurologic manifestations in IE can range from confusion to a major cerebral vascular accident. Other central nervous system complications include embolism and those that result from systemic infections such as meningitis and cerebral abscess [18]. Mycotic aneurysms also may result from vegetative emboli that lodge in intracranial, visceral, and peripheral arterial bifurcations. The mortality rate for patients who suffer intracranial aneurysms ranges from 30% to 80% [19]. The best treatment for neurologic manifestations with IE is prevention.

Embolization

Emboli form on vegetative structures and can be dislodged through valvular mechanics. These emboli then can be distributed throughout the body. Free-floating emboli lodge in arteries of the lungs, heart, bowel, spleen, and extremities. The middle cerebral artery can suffer embolic events producing central nervous system symptoms. Neurologic embolization accounts for up to 65% of all embolic events [20].

IE involving the aortic and mitral valves produces the highest rate of embolization. In IE, embolization can occur before diagnosis and may be the precipitating event for seeking health care. Embolization also may occur during or after IE intervention. Antibiotic therapy reduces the risk of embolization during the first 2 weeks of intervention [21]. Treatment of embolization may require surgical intervention to remove valve vegetation or replace severely damaged valves.

Anticoagulation therapy as treatment for embolization is controversial [22]. Generally, all anticoagulation therapy is discontinued for the first 2 weeks of antibiotic therapy in patients who have prosthetic valve *Staphylococcus aureus* IE and recent central nervous system embolization [23]. After two weeks, anticoagulation therapy is reintroduced cautiously.

The role of the critical care nurse

A thorough history to identify conditions that may predispose the patient to IE is imperative. This history will identify patients at potential risk for this devastating disease. Retrieval of historical data related to recent surgical cardiac procedures, especially prosthetic valve insertion, should be noted. Identification of signs and symptoms experienced before hospitalization will assist in verification of the IE diagnosis.

Laboratory tests are important. Blood cultures and susceptibility testing remain important mechanisms for IE diagnosis and treatment [24]. It is important for the nurse to retrieve timely blood cultures accurately for patients suspected of having IE.

Administration of bactericidal antibiotics is critical to recovery. Maintaining an administration schedule that promotes high antibiotic concentrations in the circulating bloodstream is instrumental in penetrating vegetations and killing causative bacteria. The patient should be educated to expect long-term oral or intravenous antibiotic administration after discharge.

Preventing further bacterial exposure should be incorporated into the patient's plan of care. Consistent monitoring of infusion sites should be undertaken to prevent infiltration and phlebitis. Intravenous fluids and tubing should be changed routinely, and intravenous sites should be rotated based on hospital policy.

Oral care is important to maintain integrity of the oral mucosa. It is important to keep teeth and gums healthy because these can be sites of further bacterial exposure for vegetative tissue. Periodontal disease and dental caries should be monitored. No elective oral procedures should be initiated during therapy for IE. Only critical procedures should be performed.

The nurse should work within the nursing process to address sequentially all components that promote improved health for the patient who has IE (Fig. 1). Patients who experience CHF during IE pose a challenge to critical care management. Diuretics and afterload reduction with intravenous nitroglycerine and angiotensin-converting enzyme inhibitors may be used as presurgical interventions.

Investigations in prevention and treatment

The critical care nurse should stay abreast of current research related to management of the patient who has IE. Research related to prevention and treatment of nosocomial endocarditis, prosthetic valve endocarditis, and endocarditis in intravenous drug users is ongoing, as is research on bacterium and host modifications. Modifications of prosthetic valve biomaterial properties to reduce adherence also are being researched. This

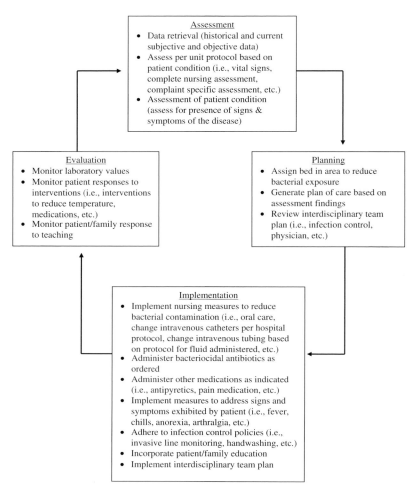

Fig. 1. Infective endocarditis management in critical care.

mechanism for preventing IE includes impregnation of biomaterial with antiseptic agents. Research related to success of this technique is ongoing [25].

Vaccines to prevent bacterial adhesion to cardiac valve leaflets are under investigation also. Vaccination against *Streptococci FimA* protein [26] and staphylococcal fibronectin-binding and collagen-binding proteins [27] have demonstrated limited success. Limitations include the quality of the host immune response.

Systemic pharmaceutical investigations includes drugs that focus on bacteriophage-encoded bacteriolytic enzymes. These molecules digest essential gram-positive peptidoglycan. They also possess antibacterial properties [28]. Results are limited in scope, but this approach demonstrates a new methodology that addresses a novel pharmaceutical mechanism of action for intervention.

The use of platelet antiaggregants to reduce vegetation formation has demonstrated limited success. Problems with antiaggregants include reduced platelet activity and increased risk of secondary bleeding. Based on these findings, antiaggregants are not currently recommended for IE management.

Summary

Most infective processes are straightforward and can be diagnosed from bacterial findings in a single test. IE does not always follow this tenet, so establishing the diagnosis can be difficult. The salient features of IE may present atypically or be obscured by the presence of preexisting and coexisting diseases. Flulike symptoms may mask the beginning of this devastating disease.

Early diagnosis of IE is important because of its high risk of morbidity and mortality. Management of the patient who has IE is complex and requires interventions by infectious disease specialists, cardiologists, respiratory therapists, and critical care nurses to address the many multifaceted complications. Early evaluation, diagnostic validation, multidisciplinary management, prompt pharmaceutical initiation, and intense critical care nursing intervention are necessary to reduce the probability of long-standing complications and to improve patient outcomes.

References

[1] Millar BC, Moore JE. Emerging issues in infective endocarditis. Emerg Infect Dis 2004;10(6):1110–6.

[2] Cabell CH, Barsic B, Bayer AS, et al. Clinical findings complications and outcomes in a large prospective study of definite endocarditis: the International Collaboration on Endocarditis—Prospective Cohort study. Abstract 22. Presented at the 7th International Symposium on Modern Concepts in Endocarditis and Cardiovascular Infections. Chamonix, France, June 26–28, 2003.

[3] Fowler VG, Miro JM, Hoen B, et al. Staphylococcus aureus endocarditis. JAMA 2005;293(24):3012–21.

[4] Baddour LM, Wilson WR, Bayer AS, et al. Infective endocarditis diagnosis, antimicrobial therapy, and management of complications. A statement for healthcare professionals from the Committee on Rheumatic Fever, Endocarditis, and Kawasaki Disease, Council on Cardiovascular Disease in the Young, and the Councils on Clinical Cardiology, Stroke and Cardiovascular Surgery and Anesthesia, American Heart Association. Circulation 2005;111: e394–433.

[5] Mylonakis E, Calderwood S. Infective endocarditis in adults. N Engl J Med 2001;345(18):1318–30.

[6] MacGregor JS, Cheitlin M. Diagnosis and management of infective endocarditis. Tex Heart Inst J 1989; 16(4):230–8.

[7] Brusch J. Infective endocarditis. 2005. Available at: http://www.emedicine.com/MED/topic671.htm. Accessed June 18, 2006.

[8] Durack DT, Lukes AT, Bright DK. New criteria for diagnosis of infective endocarditis: utilization of specific echocardiographic findings: Duke Endocarditis Service. Am J Med 1994;96:200–9.

[9] Ramsdale D, Turner-Stokes L. Prophylaxis and treatment of infective endocarditis in adults: concise guidelines. Advisory Group of the British Cardiac Society Clinical Practice Committee; 2004.

[10] Sexton DJ, Spelman D. Current best practices and guidelines assessment and management of complications in infective endocarditis. Cardiol Clin 2003;21: 273–82.

[11] Middlemost S, Wisenbaugh T, Meyerowitz C, et al. A case for early surgery in native left-sided endocarditis complicated by heart failure: results in 203 patients. J Am Coll Cardiol 1991;18:663–7.

[12] Fernicola DJ, Roberts WC. Frequency of ring abscess and cuspal infection in active infective endocarditis involving bioprosthetic valves. Am J Cardiol 1993;72:314–23.

[13] Anguera I, Miro JM, Vilacosta I, et al. Aorto-cavitary fistulous tract formation in infective endocarditis: clinical and echocardiographic features of 76 cases and risk factors for mortality. Eur Heart J 2005;26:288–97.

[14] Mullany CJ, Chua YL, Schaff HV, et al. Early and late survival after surgical treatment of culture-positive active endocarditis. Mayo Clin Proc 1995;17: 1177–82.

[15] Robinson SL, Saxe SM, Lucas CE, et al. Splenic abscess associated with endocarditis. Surgery 1992;112: 781–6.

[16] Kim HS, Cho MS, Hwang SH, et al. Splenic abscess associated with endocarditis in a patient on hemodialysis: a case report. J Korean Med Sci 2005;20:313–5. Available at: http://jkms.kams.or.kr/2005/pdf/04313. prf. Accessed April 21, 2006.

[17] Heiro M, Nikskelainen J, Engblom E, et al. Neurologic manifestations of infective endocarditis: a 17-year experience in a teaching hospital in Finland. Arch Intern Med 2000;160:2781–7.

[18] Patel FM, Das A, Banerjee AK. Neuropathological complications of infective endocarditis: study of autopsy material. Neurol India 2001;49:41–6. Available at: http://www.neurologyindia.com/article.asp?issn= 0028-3886;year=2001;volume=49;issue=1;spage=41; epage=6;aulast=Patel. Accessed April 22, 2006.

[19] Wilson WR, Giuliani ER, Danielson GK, et al. Management of complications of infective endocarditis. Mayo Clin Proc 1982;57:162–70.

[20] Omari B, Shapiro S, Ginzton L, et al. Predictive risk factors for periannular extension of native valve endocarditis: clinical and echocardiographic analyses. Chest 1989;96:1273–9.

[21] Steckelberg JM, Murphy JG, Ballard D, et al. Emboli in infective endocarditis: the prognostic value of echocardiography. Ann Intern Med 1991;114: 634–40.

[22] Salem DN, Daudelin HD, Levine HJ, et al. Antithrombotic therapy in valvular heart disease. Chest 2001;119:207S–19S.

[23] Tornos P, Almirante B, Mirabet S, et al. Infective endocarditis due to Staphylococcus aureus: deleterious effect of anticoagulant therapy. Arch Intern Med 1999;159:473–5.

[24] Moreillou P, Que YA. Infective endocarditis. Lancet 2004;363:139–49.

[25] Schaff HV, Carrel TP, Jamieson WR, et al. Para-valvular leak and other events in silzone-coated mechanical heart valves: a report from AVERT. Ann Thorac Surg 2002;73:785–92.

[26] Kitten T, Munro CL, Wang A, et al. Vaccination with FimA from Streptococcus parasanguis protect rats from endocarditis caused by other viridans streptococci. Infect Immun 2002;70:422–5.

[27] Schennings T. Immunization with fibronectin binding protein from Staphylococcus aureus protects against experimental endocarditis in rate. Microb Pathog 1993;15:227–36.

[28] Fischetti VA. Phage antibacterials make a comeback. Nat Biotechnol 2001;19:734–5.

ELSEVIER
SAUNDERS

Crit Care Nurs Clin N Am 19 (2007) 107–113

CRITICAL CARE
NURSING CLINICS
OF NORTH AMERICA

Avian Influenza: Are We Ready?

Stephen D. Krau, PhD, RN, CT[a,b,*],
Lynn C. Parsons, DSN, RN, CNA-BC[c]

[a]*School of Nursing, Vanderbilt University Medical Center, Nashville, TN, USA*
[b]*Critical Care Unit, Vanderbilt University Medical Center, Nashville, TN, USA*
[c]*School of Nursing, P.O. Box 81, Middle Tennessee State University, Murfreesboro, TN 37132, USA*

With all of the advances in health care and medicine, it would seem that we would be prepared for a pandemic such as bird flu. However, in spite of the billion dollars the United States Congress has proposed for the flu budget, only part of the solution is being addressed [1]. The threat of an H5N1 influenza virus (avian flu) pandemic is substantial, and an effective response is contingent upon effective coordination among state and local public health authorities and individual health care providers [2]. It is imperative that health care workers take an active role in the plans to meet demands that will be placed on the health care system. This is accomplished by developing an understanding of the etiology and manifestations of the virus, and becoming familiar with recent advances in research that address the demands of a pandemic. Equally important are the ethical considerations our state of preparedness will pose on the health care system, the community, and health care workers, both professionally and personally.

Critical care nurses are in a pivotal role as it relates to planning for this potential pandemic. With projections of the impact, it is important to consider what would happen if 25% to 30% of the nurses, physicians, and support staff were too sick to come to work [3,4]. A study by the Congressional Budget Office estimates several consequences of a severe pandemic. The study indicates that 200 million people in the United States could be affected, with 90 million being critically ill and 2 million dying. It is estimated that a pandemic would decrease the gross national product by 5%, and the total approximate economic cost would be approximately 675 billion dollars [4]. As of August 23, 2006, the World Health Organization has reported 241 human cases of avian flu across 10 countries, with 141 deaths. This constitutes a 58% mortality rate for identified cases [5]. The missing link to a logical pandemic spread is the lack of human-to-human transmission whereby analysis shows near all cases have resulted from direct contact with poultry, although this is not exclusive [6]. With the low probability of human-to-human contact, complacency about the potential for a pandemic is not an option. Additionally, even if H5N1 proves to have a negligible impact, planning will raise awareness and improve preparedness for a future pandemic influenza strain or another public health disaster such as smallpox, anthrax, or severe acute respiratory syndrome (SARS) [6].

It is important to consider different aspects of a pandemic before it occurs so that there is a plan of action in place. As this plan develops and evolves, it is imperative critical care nurses contribute as informed health care. This can only occur when there is a deliberate effort to understand the virus, its implications, current research, and through considering the ethical issues this pandemic could pose.

* Corresponding author. School of Nursing, Vanderbilt University Medical Center, 461 21st Ave. South, Nashville, TN 37240.
E-mail address: steve.krau@vanderbilt.edu (S.D. Krau).

Overview of the avian influenza

The avian influenza is an influenza virus that occurs naturally in many wild birds but does not usually make them sick and does not typically kill them. However, avian influenza is very contagious among birds and can cause illness in and/or kill some domesticated birds, including chickens, ducks, and turkeys. Infected birds transmit the virus in their saliva, nasal secretions, and feces.

In humans, influenza is transmitted by inhalation of infectious droplets or droplet nuclei, by direct contact, and possibly by indirect (fomite) contact, with self-inoculation to the upper respiratory tract, or mucosa of the conjunctiva [7–9]. For human influenza A(H5N1) infections, evidence to date is consistent with bird-to-human transmission, possible environment-to-human transmission, and most importantly, limited and nonsustained human-to-human transmission [9]. Because the virus has not mutated to facilitate efficient person-to-person contact since its discovery over 10 years ago, there are some who believe it will not mutate and will ultimately pose only a minimal threat. However, the H5N1 influenza virus could adapt and change as influenza viruses such as those that caused Asian influenza in 1958 and Hong Kong influenza in 1968 have done [6].

How avian influenza could become a human pandemic strain

Anatomically, each strain of influenza is named for the hemagglutinin (H) and the neuraminidase (N), which involves the subtypes. Currently, we know of 16 subtypes of hemagglutinin and 9 of nueraminidase for influenza A. Hence, the identification of strains is based on subtypes such as H5N1 [10].

There are two processes by which the current strain of avian influenza could become a human pandemic strain. Mutation is a process of evolution whereby the virus may alter its genes and antigenicity and acquire new surface antigens. These new antigens may allow the newly formed virus to bypass the human immune response. Reassortment is a synergistic process in which human flu virus and avian flu virus infect the same host simultaneously. The genes from the two strains interchange resulting in a new strain composed of genetic materials from the two original strains. The resulting virus—the new hybrid virus—possesses surface antigens that the human immune system may not recognize [10].

In addition, H5N1 avian influenza virus is not the only avian virus that has recently been found to infect humans. However, it is perceived as posing the greatest threat for a pandemic. Because the virus was only found in birds and a few other animals before 1997, the recent transmission, or "jump," from bird to human represents cause for concern.

Human-to-human transmission

Human-to-human transmission of avian influenza has been suggested in several household clusters [11], and in one case probably through child-to-mother transmission [12]. In these cases, intimate contact without the use of precautions was implicated. No cases have been clearly identified as human-to-human transmission through small particle aerosols [9,10]. Some evidence suggests that the virus may be adapting to humans, but because of the small number of cases and the geographic distributions among them, more epidemiologic and virologic studies are needed for confirmation [9].

The concern about the avian influenza virus rests in its ability to mutate or reassort. Currently the virus is considered by the World Health Organization to be in phase three of six phases of alert for pandemic classification. It is not considered pandemic because of its current inefficiency in transmission from human to human. Once this transmission is efficient and sustained, we will be in the midst of a serious pandemic [4].

There is also current evidence to support the idea that human-to-human transmission of the virus is limited because H5N1 viruses replicate effectively only in the cells of the lower respiratory tract. The avian virus receptor is prevalent only in the lowest part of the human respiratory system. This impedes the transmission of the virus as opposed to viruses that flourish in the upper respiratory tract and are transmitted easily through coughing or sneezing [13].

Environment-to-human transmission

Because the avian influenza virus is virulent, as are most type A viruses, it can survive in the environment that may prove a mode of transmission. Ingestion of water where contaminated birds have been, or conjunctival inoculation from swimming in contaminated water, are also potential modes of transmission. Additionally, places where avian feces is used as agricultural fertilizer is another possible risk.

Clinical features of persons infected with avian influenza

The clinical picture of the patient infected with avian influenza is based on descriptions of hospitalized patients. Most cases have been previously healthy young children or adults [9]. It is estimated that the incubation period of this virus is longer than for other human influenzas. Varying cases indicate this incubation period can be from 2 to 5 days and up to 8 to 17 days.

Initial symptoms of H5N1 avian influenza infection include high fever (typically over 38°F) and influenza-like symptoms primarily affecting the lower respiratory tract. Lower respiratory tract symptoms are usually evident early and are often discerned at presentation. Respiratory changes, including dyspnea, crackles, and/or respiratory distress, are common. Radiologic findings have included diffuse or multifocal infiltrates consistent with pneumonia. Diarrhea, vomiting, abdominal pain, pleuritic pain, and bleeding from oral and nasal mucosa have been reported early in the course of symptoms for some patients [9]. Diarrhea is more watery than what is seen in persons affected by human viruses, and conjunctivitis with H5N1 avian influenza is rare (although it is sometimes seen in other forms of avian influenza). Sputum production is variable and sometimes bloody [9].

In Thailand, the median time from the onset of illness to the progression of acute respiratory distress syndrome was 6 days, with a range of 4 to 13 days [14]. Multiorgan dysfunction with signs of renal failure and sometimes cardiac compromise, including cardiac dilation and supraventricular tachyarrhythmias, have been common [11,14,15]. Other complications associated with H5N1 infections have been ventilator-associated pneumonia, pulmonary hemorrhage, pneumothorax, pancytopenia, sepsis syndrome without documented bacteremia, and Reye's syndrome [9].

Management of the patient who has avian influenza

However, whereas the number of affected persons remains small and manageable, patients who have suspected or proven influenza A(H5N1) should be hospitalized [9]. In the hospital, patients can be isolated, monitored, and receive appropriate pharmacological therapy. Within 48 hours of admission to a hospital, most patients who have avian influenza A(H5N1) have required ventilatory support [11,14]. These patients have also required intensive care for multiorgan dysfunction and failure and in some cases hypotension. In addition, vigorous treatment with broad-spectrum antibiotics, antiviral agents, and, in some cases, corticosteroids have been used [9]. The efficacy of thesewarrants further study, late institution of the drugs has not had an appreciable effect on mortality rates. It seems early initiation of viral drugs produce the best outcomes [10,11,14].

Currently, two classes of drugs with antiviral properties against influenza viruses are available: inhibitors of the neuroaminidase, an enzyme on the surface of the influenza virus; and inhibitors of the ion channel activity of membrane protein on the virus. The former include amantidine and rimantidane, and the latter include oseltamivir and zanamivir [16]. The therapeutic efficacy of amantadine is unclear in human influenza because of limited studies, but there have been reductions in fever and illness by one day seen in adults and children [17]. Currently, the optimal dose and duration of treatment with neuraminidase inhibitors are uncertain. Neurotoxicity and a rapid development of drug resistance are major disadvantages of amantadine, whereas rimantidine is less neurotoxic but is not available in most parts of the world [16].

Both zanamivir and oseltamivir have proven efficacy in the treatment of human influenza when started early during the course of the illness or as a postexposure prophylaxis [14]. Zanamivir is administered through inhalation because of its poor oral availability and has been used against various human influenza viruses, but has limited use in the elderly because it may cause bronchospasm. Oseltamivir can be given orally. Drug resistance has been identified as a potential development for both of these drugs because of the mutations of the hemaglutinin or neuraminidase in the virus [16]. It is important to reiterate that data are scarce on these medications in human cases of influenza H5N1 because most of the studies have been done on animal models.

Risks for health care workers

Caring for patients who have avian influenza poses a risk to health care workers. The obvious risk is exposure to the virus, that without vaccination, people are considered universally immunologically naïve. Universal precautions with particular attention to droplet precautions are currently recommended for the care of patients infected with human influenza. Because of the uncertainty as to which modes avian influenza may first transmit between humans, additional precautions for health care workers involved in the care of patients with documented or suspected avian influenza should be instituted [18]. Health care workers should also be alert to: "patients with a history of travel within 10 days to a country with avian influenza activity and are hospitalized with a severe febrile respiratory illness, or are otherwise under evaluation for avian influenza, should be managed using isolation precautions identical to those recommended for patients with known Severe Acute Respiratory Syndrome." [18] Specific guidelines for precautions are outlined in Box 1.

Those providing care for patients who have avian influenza should monitor their temperature twice daily and report any elevations over 38°C immediately for diagnostic testing. In addition, if health care providers feel unwell for any reason, they should not be involved in direct patient care until an alternate cause is identified. If an alternative cause is not identified, they should be treated immediately with oseltamivir on the assumption of influenza infection [9].

Combination guidelines from the World Health Organization, and Center for Disease Control and Prevention indicate that for persons who have had possible exposure to infectious aerosols, secretions, excretions, or other body fluids due to a lapse in aseptic technique, consideration for postexposure prophylaxis is appropriate with oseltamivir for 7 to 10 days at 75 mg once a day [9]. Health care workers involved in high-risk procedures should also be considered for pharmacologic prophylaxis [9,10]. However, as with new strains of bacteria, there is a risk of promoting the emergence of neuraminidase inhibitor-resistant viruses. As such, the indiscriminate use of these drugs should be discouraged [19].

In addition, current recommendations from the Center for Disease Control and Prevention indicate health care workers involved in the care of patients who have documented or suspected avian influenza should be vaccinated with the most recent seasonal human influenza vaccine. This not only provides protection against the predominant circulating influenza strain, but also will reduce the likelihood of a health care worker being co-infected with human and avian strains, whereby genetic rearrangement (reassortment) could take place, leading to the emergence of potential pandemic strain [18].

Box 1. Precautions for health care workers engaged in the care of persons suspected to be infected with avian influenza (H1N5)

Standard precautions
1. Engage in hand hygiene before and after all patient contact or contact with items potentially contaminated with respiratory secretions [18]

Contact precautions
2. Use gloves and gown for all direct patient contact
3. Use dedicated equipment such as stethoscopes, disposable blood pressure cuffs, disposable thermometers, and so forth [18]

Eye protection (ie, goggles or face shields)
4. Wear when within 3 feet of the patient [18]

Airborne precautions
5. Place the patient in an airborne isolation room. Such rooms should have monitored negative air pressure in relation to corridor, with 6 to 12 air changes per hour and exhaust air directly outside or have recirculated air filtered by a high-efficiency particulate air filter; if an airborne isolation room is unavailable, contact the health care facility engineer to assist or use portable high-efficiency particulate air filters to augment the number of ACH [18]
6. Use a fit-tested respirator, at least as protective as a National Institute of Occupational Safety and Health-approved N-95 filtering facepiece (ie, disposable) respirator) when entering the room [18]

Visitors
7. Educate and limit number of visitors

Current status on vaccine for avian influenza

Although there is currently no commercially available vaccine to protect humans against H5N1 virus that is being seen in Asia and Europe, there are studies underway. An experimental vaccine for avian influenza (H5N1) was produced from a seed of a virus isolated in Vietnam. Treanor and colleagues [20] studied an experimental vaccine in detail and conclude that it is possible to generate immunity with the "use of a purified, subviron vaccine administered in two relatively high doses." The immunogenicity threshold for this study was set at an antibody titer of 1:40 or greater, which is typically thought of as seroprotective. Each of these two doses is six times the dose that is used in standard influenza immunizations. The experimental doses were found to induce immune responses in about half of the adults tested. The researchers suggest that there may be some dose-sparring approaches to enhance the efficacy of the vaccine. There have been several small studies that demonstrate the use of adjuvants such as aluminum [21], or the intradermal administration of the vaccine [22,23], as opposed to the typical intramuscular injection of influenza vaccines. An adjuvant that has been also found effective in influenza vaccination is an oil-based compound called MF-59, a compound primarily composed of squalene [24]. Additionally, recent demonstration of an experimental vaccine shows a substantial increase in immune response when administered to subjects 16 months after the initial priming series [24].

Pharmaceutical companies are reluctant to enter or remain in the production of vaccines. Unpredictable consumer demands coupled with lack of financial incentives make the production of vaccines somewhat risky. Currently the worldwide manufacturing capacity for influenza vaccine is estimated at 900 million doses at the dose level of 15 μg. Clearly with the requirement of two doses at 90 μg per person, only 75 million persons—less than 1.5% of the world's population—could be fully immunized [4]. Based on the preliminary studies, only half of those would achieve seroprotection and it is not known whether this vaccine will offer cross-protection against other H5N1 strains of influenza. It is probable that more than one H5N1 vaccine will be needed.

There are live attenuated vaccines that are being developed that would produce more antibodies after one injection and would have several other advantages over inactivated vaccines in a pandemic [25]. One of the major disadvantages could be the reassortment of a virus if the vaccine is given too early. A reassorted virus could introduce the pandemic virus into the population.

There is discussion about a staged vaccine program. Once available and instituted, a maximum effect on reducing transmission of avian influenza would occur if children are vaccinated first, whereby school children have the highest rates of influenza transmission. The lowest impact on transmission will occur if elderly are vaccinated first [26].

Ethical considerations for an influenza pandemic

There is no certainty of an avian influenza (H5N1) pandemic. There are those who think the planning, thought, and finances that have gone into the potential for an avian influenza pandemic are pointless. However, the proposition is one that is "all or nothing" [1]. Who could have predicted the AIDS/HIV epidemic? There were fewer "warning signs" for AIDS than what we have seen historically with influenza epidemics. It stands to reason that overreacting will have a more beneficial effect in the long run on the health care system's ability to serve most of the people in the world, rather than to ignore the lessons of history. It is important not only to know of the current state of avian influenza (H5N1), the current research on vaccines, and the current recommendations, but also to consider the ethics of health care as it relates to this potential pandemic.

Ethical issues that would come to prominence during such a pandemic would involve surveillance issues, quarantine issues, resource allocation, justice, and issues of personal choice for health care workers [1]. These are core problems that will emerge in a pandemic that warrant careful consideration before the occurrence.

In our mobile society, surveillance is an important issue. This requires a system to detect and respond to the reports of an avian influenza outbreak so that supplies can be given to ameliorate the situation. Although the World Health Organization predicts the outbreak will occur in Asia, we must remain vigilant worldwide. There is a fine balance between surveillance and intrusiveness that has been demonstrated by the myriad sexually transmitted diseases and other diseases. Issues of privacy will be particularly salient, particularly in an environment of fear and mass communication.

Quarantine procedures will need to be put in place at the first local outbreak of a pandemic to prevent the spread and amplification of the disease [1]. This poses numerous questions about who, where, how long, and what circumstances. Although there are recommendations in place from the Centers for Disease Control and

Prevention, there are many questions about who will enforce this quarantine: what will the effect be of potential pandemonium, and what of work loss or financial loss of the individual who is quarantined? The questions are extensive but warrant consideration.

Resource allocation is an issue in any crisis. Vaccine policy is driven larger by politics, in which vaccinations are given by categories or vulnerability rather than efficacy [1]. Who should receive vaccinations? What principles of justice guide these decisions? As stated by Zoloth and Zoloth [1], "Epidemics force us toward utilitarian conclusions, justifying the distribution schemes that favor the most useful over the neediest, so the most useful can best serve the overall telos of a functioning society." Is this acceptable to the people of the United States, or the world? Allocation schemes pose inherent values. For example, look at the issue when anthrax prophylaxis was given to members of Congress before postal workers.

Additionally consider the increase in volume and expenses for not only pharmaceutical but also other supplies such as gowns, masks, and gloves. Consider how in the midst of the pandemic, supports from social service agencies and public services would be limited. Lastly, what occurs when all local hospitals are closed to new admissions? These questions should lead to practical planning for any health care institution.

Probably the most difficult question for critical care nurses and for most health care workers will be that of personal duty. An avian influenza pandemic would bring about a moral dilemma for health care workers in their competing roles as professionals versus family members [1]. Some states regard the obligation to treat during an emergency as a legal duty with criminal sanctions for those who refuse.

SARS provides a recent prototype of an example whereby the issue of personal duty has been demonstrated. A study involving 15,025 health care workers from nine major health care institutions in Singapore during a 2003 SARS epidemic yields results that might have implications for predictions in the event of an influenza epidemic [27]. Although personal risk was identified by 76% of the respondents, panic can be avoided by the implementation of simple protective measures based on sound hygiene and epidemiologic principles. This study, along with a study by Bournes and Ferguson-Pare' [28] in the wake of a Toronto outbreak of SARS, focuses on principles that might ameliorate the personal affect that a comparable avian influenza outbreak might have on health care workers.

Summary

We cannot be certain when the next influenza pandemic will emerge, or even whether it will be caused by avian influenza (H5N1) or some unrelated virus. However, we can be certain that an influenza pandemic will occur [29]. The United States is leading the scientific effort to contain the pandemic through vaccine studies and antiviral studies. The need for pandemic influenza preparedness is extensive and expensive. Planning entails increased development of antivirals and vaccines, effective surveillance systems not only for people, but in agriculture, effective communication systems, plans to continue essential services, identification of health care priorities, and thorough guidelines for care. Critical care nurses, as well as all health care professionals, need to consider where their personal and professional obligations meet and end. There should already be discussions of contingency plan of the institution in which they are employed and the community in which they live. Additionally, a personal plan for their families with regard to economics, safety, and optimizing personal health outcomes during such a crisis should be considered. As many have said, "It is not a matter of if, but rather of when." Although the pandemic might not be the avian flu, history has taught us that pandemics surface with little warning and can have devastating effects on human lives, and can over tax the already fragile health care system.

References

[1] Zoloth L, Zoloth S. Don't be chicken: bioethics and avian flu. Am J Bioeth 2006;6(1):5–8.

[2] Barnitz L, Berkwits M. The health care response to pandemic influenza. Ann Intern Med 2006;145(2): 135–7.

[3] Anderson E. Avian flu—are you prepared to fight a pandemic? AAOHN J 2006;54(1):8–10.

[4] Poland G. Vaccines against avian influenza—a race against time. N Engl J Med 2006;354(13):1411–3.

[5] World Health Organization. Avian influenza. Cumulative number of confirmed human cases of avian influenza A/(H5N1) reported to the WHO. Available at: http://www.who.int/csr/disease/avian_influenza/country/cases_table_2006_08_23/en/index.html. Accessed September 30, 2006.

[6] Bartlett J. Planning for avian influenza. Ann Intern Med 2006;145(2):141–9.

[7] Salgado CD, Farr BM, Hall KK, et al. Influenza in the acute hospital setting. Lancet Infect Dis 2002;2: 145–55 [Erratum, Lancet Infect Dis 2002;2:283].

[8] Bridges CB, Kuehnert MJ, Hall CB. Transmission of influenza: implications for control in health care settings. Clin Infect Dis 2003;37:1094–101.

[9] Beigel JH, Farrar J, Han AM, et al. Avian influenza A (H5N1) infections in humans. N Engl J Med 2005; 353:1374–85.

[10] Jin XW, Mossad SB. Avian influenza: an emerging pandemic threat. Cleve Clin J Med 2005;12(72): 1129–34.

[11] Hien TT, Liem NT, Dung NT, et al. Avian influenza A (H5N1) in 10 patients in Viet Nam. N Engl J Med 2004;350:1179–88.

[12] Ungchosak K, Auewarakul P, Dowell SF, et al. Probably person to person transmission of avian influenza A (H5N1). N Engl J Med 2005;352:333–40.

[13] Kyoko S, Ebina M, Yamada S, et al. Influenza virus receptors in the human airway. Nature 2006; 440(7083):435–6.

[14] Chotpitayasunonduh T, Ungchusak K, Hanshaoworakul W, et al. Human disease from influenzae A (H5N1), Thailand 2004. Emerg Infect Dis 2005; 11:201–9.

[15] Chan PK. Outbreak of avian influenza A(H5N1) virus infection in Hong Kong in 1997. Clin Infect Dis 2002;34(Suppl 2):S58–64.

[16] de Jong MD, Hien TT. Avian influenza A (H5N1). J Clin Virol 2006;35(1):2–13.

[17] Nicholson KG, Wood JM, Zambon M. Influenza. Lancet 2003;362:1733–45.

[18] Center for Disease Control and Prevention. Interim recommendations for infection control in health-care facilities caring for patients with known or suspected avian influenxa. Available at: http://www.cdc.gov/flu/avian/professional/infect-control.htm. Accessed October 12, 2006.

[19] Wong SS, Yuen K. Avian influenza virus infections in humans. Chest 2006;129(1):156–68.

[20] Treanor JJ, Campbell JD, Zangwill KM, et al. Safety and immunogenicity of an inactivated subvirion influenza A (H5N1) vaccine. N Engl J Med 2006;354(13):1343–51.

[21] Hehme N, Engelmann HJ, Kuenzel W. Immunogenecity of a monovalent aluminum-adjuvanted influenza whole virus vaccine for pandemic use. Virus Res 2004;103:163–71.

[22] Belshe RB, Newman FK, Cannon J, et al. Serum antibody responses after intradermal vaccination against influenza. N Engl J Med 2004;351:2286–94.

[23] Kenney RT, Frech SA, Muenz LR, et al. Dose sparring with intradermal injection of influenza vaccine. N Engl J Med 2004;351:2295–301.

[24] Stephenson I, Nicholson KG, Colegate A, et al. Boosting immunity to influenza H5N1 with MF59-adjuvanted H5N3 A/Duck/Singapore 97 vaccine in a primed human population. Vaccine 2003;21:1687–93.

[25] Monto AS. Vaccines and antiviral drugs in pandemic preparedness. Emerg Infect Dis 2006;12(1): 55–60.

[26] Ferguson NM, Cummings DA, Fraser C, et al. Strategies for mitigating an influenza pandemic. Nature 2006;442(7107):448–52.

[27] Koh D, Lim MK, Chia SE, et al. Risk perceptions and impact of severe acute respiratory syndrome (SARS) on work and personal lives of health care workers in Singapore: what can we learn? Med Care 2005;43(7):676–82.

[28] Bournes DA, Ferguson-Pare' M. Persevering through a difficult time during the SARS outbreak in Toronto. Nurs Sci Q 2005;18(4):324–33.

[29] Fauci AS. Pandemic influenza threat and preparedness. Emerg Infect Dis 2006;12(1):73–7.

ELSEVIER
SAUNDERS

Crit Care Nurs Clin N Am 19 (2007) 115–120

CRITICAL CARE
NURSING CLINICS
OF NORTH AMERICA

Index

Note: Page numbers of article titles are in **boldface** type.

A

Acute-phase proteins, in inflammatory response, 3, 5

Acyclovir (Zovirax), 49–50

Amantadine, for avian influenza, 109

Amblyomma americanum (Lone Star tick), 31
 Southern tick-associated rash illness from, 41

American dog tick (*Dermacentor variabilis*), 28–30
 Rocky Mountain spotted fever and, 28–30, 32

Aminoglycosides, 47

Amphotericin B (Amphocin), 49

Ampicillin (Principen), 45

Ampicillin/sulbactam (Unasyn), 45

Anaplasma phagocytophilia, in human monocytotrophic ehrlichiosis, 34

Antifungals, 49

Antigens, in immune response, 10

Antimicrobial resistance, **53–60**
 antimicrobial management and, combination therapy, 55–56
  guidelines and protocols for, 55, 57
  multidisciplinary team in, 56
  nursing process approach to, 58
  rotation of, 56
 costs of, 54
 factors in, 53
 hand hygiene and, 57
 infection and, 54–55
 nursing responsibilities and, 56–58
 organisms in, 53–54
 skin surface integrity and, 57
 surveillance of patterns in, 56–58

Antimicrobial(s), aminoglycosides, 47
 antifungals, 49
 antivirals, 49–50
 β-lactam, 44–45

carbapenems, 46
cephalosporins, 45–46
classification of, **43–51**
clindamycin, 48
dalfopristin/quinupristin, 48–49
fluoroquinolones, 47
ketolides, 47
linezolid, 48
macrolides, 47–48
monobactams, 46–47
vancomycin hydrochloride, 48

Antivirals, 49–50
 for avian influenza, 109

Aspergillus species, in infective endocarditis, 100

Autoimmune disease pathophysiology, 11

Autoimmunity, infection and, 12

Avian influenza, **107–113**
 in birds, 107–108
 ethical considerations for pandemic, 107, 111–112
 healthcare workers and, moral dilemma of personal duty, 112
  precautions for, 110
  risks for, 109–110
 human influenza vaccination and, 110
 in humans, 109–110
 transmission of, birds-to-humans, 108
  environment-to-human, 108
  humans-to-human, 108
 vaccine for, current status of, 110–111

Aztreonam (Azactam), 46–47

B

Babesiosis, 34

Bacteremia, nosocomial enterococcal, 69

Bacteria, classification of, color, 22
 gram-positive, gram-negative, 22
 oxygen use by, 22

Moving?

Make sure your subscription moves with you!

To notify us of your new address, find your **Clinics Account Number** (located on your mailing label above your name), and contact customer service at:

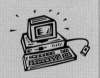

E-mail: elspcs@elsevier.com

800-654-2452 (subscribers in the U.S. & Canada)
407-345-4000 (subscribers outside of the U.S. & Canada)

Fax number: 407-363-9661

Elsevier Periodicals Customer Service
6277 Sea Harbor Drive
Orlando, FL 32887-4800

*To ensure uninterrupted delivery of your subscription, please notify us at least 4 weeks in advance of move.